Food As Medicine

Traditional Chinese Medicine-Inspired Healthy Eating Principles with Action Guide, Worksheet, and 10-Week Meal Plan to Restore Health, Beauty, and Mind

TRACY HUANG

Disclaimer

Please note that I am NOT a medical doctor; and make no claims to be. The information provided in this book is provided for general information purposes; and does not constitute medical, legal or other professional advice on any subject matter. The author of this book does not accept any responsibility for any loss which may arise from reliance on information contained within this book or on any associated websites or blogs.

Contents

Introduction

When I first came to the US in 2010 from China, the first cultural shock came to me was sitting in class and overwhelmed by the active participations of my American classmates, as in China we were taught to obey. When I was at school in China, whenever teachers asked questions, we students would immediately look down with our eyes gazing on the desk surface or on the floor, hoping teachers would not discover our presence (thankfully, I feel much more comfortable and confident in expressing my thoughts right now). The second thing I felt so different was the gap between how the American and people from my hometown consume foods.

I come from a city called Shenzhen which is south of China and close to Hong Kong. Growing up, I was always taught by my mom about how a particular food will benefit a particular part of the body. For example, she would say to me: "have some mung bean soup for your breakouts", or "drink chrysanthemum tea for your sore throat". But in the US, it seems to me that people here talk in a different food language.

In my first year in the US, I slowly put aside what I learned in China (as I didn't have my mom physically nearby to remind me of what to eat), and followed an American diet. My skin suddenly started to break out constantly without control.

A year later, I cut out wheat and dairy, which means no cow's milk, cereals, or yogurts. Then, my skin started to clear up, though not entirely.

Realizing foods could make a huge difference on my skin while being frustrated about my skin not being able to be completely cleared up, I started to explore more dietary solutions; this naturally led me back to the eating culture I grew up with in China.

While doing research, I came across Amazon Bestseller *The Beauty Detox Solutions (http://bit.ly/beauty-detox-solutions)* by nutritionist Kimberly Snyder and was grateful for reading this book, because it introduced me to the world of nutrition and green smoothies.

Although, as I study more about Traditional Chinese Medicine and Chinese food therapy, I may not fully agree with her nutritional approach, the book definitely has inspired me to scientifically understand how the stomach digests foods and the theory of food combination, consume green drinks and smoothies, and live an eating-clean lifestyle.

The therapeutic part of food is rarely talked about. As I learn more about food – one of the greatest gifts that Mother Nature gives us, the human body, and the philosophy behind Chinese food therapy, I feel that the western world should also be introduced to this missing piece in the knowledge of food (nature's gift should equally benefit all human-beings), in order to help people fully benefit from whole foods and achieve optimal state of health and well-being.

That's why I wrote this book:

It is about digging deeper into the therapeutic aspects in foods that you may not have heard of yet; it is also about choosing to eat with consciousness and exploring how food can serve as medicine to help heal the body; most importantly, it is about deepening the relationship with your own body, because you cannot improve health unless you understand your body and know what to pick accordingly to strengthen health, slow down aging process, deal with health concerns, and prevent diseases your body is prone to.

Yes, this book helps you kick off your journey to achieving all of the benefits mentioned above.

This book is a collection and summary of my personal experience with Traditional Chinese Medicine and experiments based on the teaching of Chinese Food Therapy, what I learned from my Chinese doctor, Fang-Tsuey Lin, Licensed Acupuncturist who has been practicing since 2001 in Lexington, Massachusetts, as well as key insights from a series of books written by Traditional Chinese Medicine practitioners.

Specifically, you will learn:
- What is Food Therapy after all?
- Where do these dietary ideas come from?
- Why is it different from other dietary approaches you have heard of?
- How can it help restore your health, beauty, and mind?
- How can you get started, so that you don't get lost in the wealth of knowledge (I include this part in Chapter 4, Chapter 5, and Chapter 6 because I want to help you turn knowledge into action)?

Last but not least, as I am constantly learning more about Chinese Food Therapy and may update this book in the future. If you wish to get free updates about this book, please feel free to subscribe to my mailing list: bit.ly/signup-for-bonuses.

By doing so, you will *also* be receiving:
- A Bonus Chapter that helps you understand your own body and how to find the right foods that fit only your body type,
- A individualized self-assessment sheet to help you find out your own body type in less than five minutes,
- A printable work plan to help you slowly transition from your current diet routine to TCM-inspired lifestyle,
- A printable worksheet to help you turn what you learn in this book into specific action items,
- My personal insights, experiments, and learnings on Traditional Chinese Medicine and Food Therapy along the way.

Without further ado, let's begin the journey right now!

Chapter 1: Introduction to Chinese Food Therapy

Chinese food therapy, also known as Chinese dietary therapy or nutrition therapy, is a mode of eating based on ancient Chinese people's understandings of the effects of food on the human organism. More than 4,000 years ago the Chinese discovered that food can offer therapeutic benefits apart from nutrition, and that human beings can selectively choose and consume certain foods to prevent or deal with various health conditions and to improve overall physical and physiological well-being.

Specifically speaking, Traditional Chinese Medicine therapists believe that each type of food has its own unique property which perform certain functions and can work on a particular part of the body. For example, goji berries help improve vision, whereas white radishes nourish the lungs. Hence, what you put into your mouth can directly have impacts on your body from the inside.

Therefore, following principles from Chinese food therapy can be seen as a process to improve your health and well-being by learning how to select the right foods with the right kind of therapeutic properties you need for your body.

History of Chinese Food Therapy

People had already discovered therapeutic benefits of foods as early as Xia Dynasty (2,000 BC – 1,600 BC). Back then, people already knew things like how ginger is able to not only warm up the body, but also protect it from winds and cold weathers.

Then, very basic therapeutic diets started to appear in Shang Dynasty (1,700 BC – 1,100 BC), which was around the time that soup was invented.

In Zhou Dynasty (1,100 BC – 221 BC), people became very knowledgeable with therapeutic diets while advocating the combination of five flavors from natural foods (sour, sweet, bitter, pungent and salty) as well as whole grains for healing purposes. During these times, the court would appoint a *shiyi* (similar to a nutritionist nowadays) to the palace to examine food properties, how much of each type of food to consume each time, how to combine different types of food to maximize the amount of nutritional intake, and their effects on health.

Shiyi, literally known as a dietary doctor, was regarded as the most respected profession among all types of doctors in that era. As you can imagine, people in ancient China really paid a lot of emphasis on the therapeutic aspects of foods for healing and nourishing the body. Another notable mention in late Zhou Dynasty is *Huangdi Neijing*, or *Yellow Emperor's Inner Canon*. It is probably the most important ancient Chinese medical text that has been treated as the foundational doctrine for the entire practice of Chinese medicine. The book speaks highly of the benefits of dietary therapy and has established a solid foundation for the study of Chinese food therapy.

In Han Dynasty (about 202 BC - 220), *Shen Nong Ben Cai Jing*, literally known as *The Classics of Materia Medica by Shen Nong*, was the earliest text on pharmacology in China, was written during the Han Dynasty, and featured more than 50 types of food that could be served for medicinal purposes to fight against certain ailments.

Many of other famous and influential texts on food therapy emerged during Sui Tang Dynasty (581 - 618). In his book *Qian Jin Yao Fang*, literally translated as *Prescription Worth a Thousand Gold* and regarded as the earliest medical text in China with clinical records, Sun Simiao mentioned a doctor should understand the root cause of a disease and first prescribe food as a therapy for the patients. It is only when food therapies do not work on patients that a doctor would instead prescribe medicines to them.

Additionally, in that era, another book worth mentioning is *Shi Liao Ben Cao*, literally meaning *Materia Medica on Foods*. It was the first book in China that created a comprehensive list of the therapeutic benefits of 261 foods.

As this knowledge was handed down from predecessors, it became very common to see food treated as a type of medicine in countless other medical texts that followed over the centuries. For example, *Sheng Ji Zong Lu*, literally known as *General Records of Holy Universal Relief*, is a medical text from Song Dynasty (960 -- 1279). There is a whole chapter inside the book solely dedicated to discussing dietary therapies to treat different types of ailments.

During the Ming Dynasty (1368-1644), the concept of using food therapy to achieve an optimal state of health and well-being flourished and played an even more important role in Chinese people's everyday lives. One of the most important texts is *Ben Cao*

Gang Mu (or, *Compendium of Materia Medica*) by Li Shizhen. In the book, he recorded more than 300 kinds of herbs derived from whole grains, vegetables and fruits, and more than 400 kinds from animals.

Key Philosophies Practiced by Chinese Food Therapy

By now you have learned how *Huangdi Neijing* (or, *Yellow Emperor's Inner Canon*) has served as an important doctrinal source for the practice of Chinese food therapy. In other words, Chinese dietary therapy reflects and follows the key principles of this text.

Now we are about to discuss two important concepts expressed in this medical text and how these two key beliefs are rooted in the practice of food therapy.

First, to seek great health, you should look for internal guidance. In other words, *Huangdi Neijing* believes that your first step to great health is to start from focusing on what is inside of you.

Specifically, you will need the skills of self-observation and internal awareness of the body. Self-observation means you should understand your own body including how different organs function and how blood circulates. Improving internal conditions means you should know how to take actions to promote qi blood circulation and nourish innate organs, so as to achieve vibrant health and longevity.

Because of this fundamental belief, you should start from understanding the body and yourself before determining what to eat.

Second, you should also seek external guidance. That is, you need to stay in harmony with nature and eat accordingly. *Huangdi Neijing* sees that human beings are living as a part of nature, and are thus attuned to nature's changes. Seasonal or other environmental fluctuations may cause the body to function slightly differently and to be prone to different diseases during different times.

This, then, requires you adjust your lifestyle to meet with those changes such as paying attention to both what to eat and how to eat different foods. For example, Chinese medicine recommends you consume foods with cooling properties in the hot summer such as water melons, mung bean soup, and bitter melons to remove excess heat in the body; whereas in the fall you can consider having white radishes and pears to nourish the lungs when you feel the dryness of the season.

How Chinese Food Therapy Is Different

So, now you understand some of the basics of Chinese food therapy, so here is a recap of how I feel it is different from other types of diets. In total, there are three areas that make this dietary therapy unique:

First and foremost, Chinese medicine believes that everybody is unique. So, there is no (and should be no) generic nutritional advice. That means it is not recommended that everybody follow the same particular diet. Instead, you should first take some time to understand your body before seeking any nutritional advice.

Here is an example of how everybody is born with a unique body type: one person might have cold hands and feet as long as she is exposed to air conditioning in the hot summer even when she wears enough clothes, while another person has very warm hands and feet even during the cold winter time. In that case, it is actually not good for one who often experiences cold hands and feet to have salads all the time or completely go on a raw food diet because of her special body type. Otherwise, she may become even more afraid of being exposed to cold environments.

Therefore, the best way to start looking for what's healthy to eat is to begin with identifying your unique body constitution.

The next thing that makes Chinese food therapy different from other diets is that it recognizes how foods themselves have their own unique properties and therapeutic benefits, which are different from nutritional values like vitamins and proteins and can be used to treat certain minor illnesses and other conditions. For example, you could try bitter melons to relieve constipation. Or, you could enjoy the same melon, or try some mung beans, to help heal eczema or acne.

Ancient Chinese see that whenever you bring foods into the body, it is an opportunity to heal and improve health. So, foods are more than just sustenance; they also add fuels to the machine called the human body to function more powerfully.

The third and last area that makes Chinese food therapy stand out is its belief in staying in harmony with nature. Specifically speaking, what you choose to eat and how you consume foods are subject to changes in external environments like the switch between seasons; and you should follow a routine that's based on your internal biological clock as well, which I will explain in Chapter 2.

Traditional Chinese Medicine sees that everything in this world is interconnected and interrelated. Take the example of how your body's health conditions may react to seasonal changes:

As fall comes, the temperature starts to drop and you may start to feel dryness on your skin. If you don't take care of your body properly during this season, you can develop upper respiratory infections and other lung-related problems. That's why it is particularly important to nourish the lungs by consuming the right kinds of foods like pears and lily bulbs to keep the body hydrated when the weather gets dry.

Learning how to eat right and nourish the body strategically in different seasons is one of the key practices in Chinese dietary therapy. In Chapter 2, we will explore further the techniques about functional eating in different seasons.

I hope this helps you realize that foods can indeed serve as medicine. Chinese realized thousands of years ago that foods and medicine are originated from the same source. There isn't a clear-cut line in between these two topics. When you experience any discomfort or other health conditions, foods should always be considered – as they are the greatest gifts from Mother Nature. Therefore, consider what you're putting into your body as a factor before you go out and try conventional medicine (like antibiotics for breakouts, which I don't recommend).

Side notes: to learn more about why antibiotics are bad for your acne, you may check out my post here: http://bit.ly/avoid-antibiotics.

Authority and Scientific Proof and Experts' Views on Chinese Food Therapy

As more people are getting frustrated by conventional medical treatments, more and more people are turning to alternative medicines for solutions. These days, Traditional Chinese Medicine is gaining more attention and recognition internationally.

For example, Dr. Andrew Weil, who is an American medical doctor, naturopath, advocate on holistic health, and founder of the Arizona Center for Integrative Medicine at the University of Arizona, has been a longtime proponent of TCM to treat a wide range of conditions. In fact, he even believes that it is rare that a condition *cannot* be aided via TCM, at least as an adjunctive therapy.

I am not saying that Traditional Chinese Medicine is better than conventional medicine. Nor do I have the intention to make such a statement. But I do believe that Traditional Chinese Medicine can serve as an important complementary therapy in the health care system in the west.

A 2010 study published in the National Institute of Health has proved my point. The study was conducted among 85 hypertensive patients over a period of 16 weeks; and showed that Chinese dietary therapy is "beneficial in controlling blood pressure in hypertensive patients". This study also concluded that Chinese dietary therapy "should be a component of nursing education and health education".

Another study was published in 2011 on the effectiveness of Chinese therapeutic food on regulating female reproductive hormones. Results showed that the use of Chinese kiwi fruit extract could benefit women with peri-menopausal symptoms or diseases associated with hormone disorders.

Because of both the long history of this ancient therapeutic practice and its credibility backed by authorities and multiple research studies, I'm convinced that the richness of the value it delivers can help you achieve a lot of health benefits.

So, what are these health benefits exactly? Let's dig deeper in what kinds of benefits you will enjoy from Chinese food therapy.

What Are the Benefits?

There are many great benefits to dietary therapy. For instance, dietary therapy can be implemented as preventative medicine. That's because TCM is more than just solutions you go to when you feel sick; what's amazing to me is that TCM is also a type of *mindset or mentality* that serves as reference on how to live everyday life to constantly improve your state of health and well-being. As you can tell from its philosophy, the methodologies behind Chinese dietary therapy are about encouraging these principles to be installed into your daily life.

This includes understanding your own body before choosing what's good for you to eat, studying food properties and their therapeutic benefits before deciding the most suitable options that can help heal the body, and eating different foods in different seasons. That's what makes food therapy a powerful preventative medicine – when you always eat the right food that your body needs and loves, you will greatly lower your chances of getting sick.

In modern China, many people are also using it for other purposes like weight loss, skin care and hair care. That should not be a surprise, because Chinese food therapy – a branch of Traditional Chinese Medicine – sees everything is connected. If you take care of the body internally, your skin and hair will be naturally taken care of. Slowly but surely, skin will radiate; and hair will shine.

What's more, by following a Chinese food therapy, you learn to follow the law of nature and start to understand more about how to respect your body. As a reward for taking care of the body by giving what it needs, you may experience another great benefit; the slowing down of the aging process. The secret to anti-aging is actually simple – it is to listen to your body's subtle calling and respond by giving what it needs, which is the topic we focus on in the next chapter.

As I was doing research, I found that the average life span for a Chinese living in ancient times was about 57 years old (disregarding the very high infant mortality rate in those days). However, Sun Simiao (581 -- 682) – creator of the earliest medical text in China with clinical records called *Qian Jin Yao Fang* (or, *Prescription Worth a Thousand Gold*) – lived for over 100 years! He is the one I mentioned earlier who suggested doctors recommend food therapies to patients before prescribing medicine to them. By placing great emphasis on food therapies his entire life; not only for his patients but also for himself, Sun gave a great example of how Chinese food therapy allows people to enjoy vibrant health and longevity.

So far, you've learned about the dietary history of Chinese food therapy, its two core beliefs, three key areas that make it unique, the fact that it is gaining more popularity and getting more and more science-backed, and a list of benefits that I have just discussed with you. For the next part of the book, I am excited to explore more details of Chinese food therapy with you. Coming up, I've tried my best to summarize major concepts of this 5,000-year-old practice in just one chapter.

How does it make you feel when you know the secrets to an optimal state of health and well-being, great skin with natural glow from within, shiny hair and longevity can all be found as you turn to the next page?

Chapter 2: Chinese Food Therapy

Understand These Five Food Properties

While a western diet measures nutritional value from foods by using the proper amounts of minerals, vitamins, proteins, carbohydrates and fats, Chinese food therapy attempts to understand foods and their nutritional value from their flavors, energies and actions – which is how foods act on different organs inside the body.

Before we go into details about specific principles to follow in Chinese dietary therapy, it is important to understand these four concepts to help you better grasp all of the principles recommended later on.

The Five Flavors of Foods

These five flavors include sour, bitter, sweet, pungent and salty. The concept of food flavors is important in a Chinese diet, because Chinese medicine believes that different flavors play different important roles in nourishing their respective internal organs. Specifically, foods with a sour taste act on the liver and gall bladder; with a bitter taste on the heart and small intestine; with a sweet flavor on the spleen and stomach; with a pungent flavor on the lungs and large intestine; and with a salty taste on the kidneys and bladder.

Additionally, different flavors can have their own respective benefits in terms of treating different health conditions and promoting overall health as well. Below is an overview of how different flavors can benefit you from different angles:

Sour foods (e.g. lemon and plum) can obstruct movements and, therefore, can create diarrhea and excessive perspiration; foods with bitter flavors (e.g. bitter melons, lettuce, and broccoli rabe) can reduce body heat, dry body fluid, and induce diarrhea; sweet foods (sweet potatoes, butternut squash, and beets) can help slow down acute symptoms and neutralize the toxic effects of other foods; foods that taste pungent (e.g. ginger, garlic, and onions) can induce perspiration and promote energy circulation; at last, salty foods (e.g. kelp and seaweed) can soften hardness and, therefore, could be used for treating tuberculosis of the lymph nodes and other symptoms involving the hardening of muscles or glands.

Of course, there are times when you encounter some foods with a very light flavor or little taste. Usually, these kind of foods can promote urination and may be used as diuretics. Take the example of Chinese barleys (also known as Job's tears).

Examples of foods arranged by their different flavors are listed in "Appendix B: Foods of Five Flavors".

The Five Colors of Foods

These five colors derived from nature are: green, red, yellow, white and black. Just like five flavors of foods, these five colors also act on their responding organs: green foods act on the liver and gall bladder; red on heart and small intestine; yellow on the spleen and stomach; white on the lungs and large intestine; and black on the kidneys and bladder.

20

Green foods (e.g. kales, broccoli rabe, and spinach) are especially good for detoxifying the liver and alkalizing the body; they can help the stomach and spleen better digest and absorb nutrients as well. Besides, green foods are also a great source of calcium and fiber.

Red foods (e.g. red beans, dates, and cherries) are usually rich in iron which can help alleviate anemia; they can also relieve fatigue, keep the body warm, brighten up the skin, speed up skin cell renewal process and slow down aging in skin.

Yellow foods (e.g. corns, squash, and sweet potatoes) contain beta-carotene, riboflavin and other nutrients that can help prevent heart diseases and cancer, cleanse blood and improve skin.

White foods such as pears, lily bulbs and white radish are good for nourishing the lungs and skin. These foods are especially good for the fall when the weather is very dry.

As for black foods (e.g. black beans, black rice, and black sesame seeds), they are rich in proteins and minerals and contain a lot of health benefits that nourish the skin and the kidneys, strengthen the heart, lower blood sugar levels, slow down the aging process and promote longevity.

Examples of foods arranged by their different colors are listed in "Appendix C: Foods of Five Colors".

The Five Energies of Foods

The five energies of foods are cold, cool, neutral, warm and hot. But these adjectives – "cold", "cool", neutral "," warm and hot– do not refer to the present states of foods, or the actual temperatures of the foods that you can feel. Instead, they measure the energies given to the body from inside after the foods are digested.

Ancient Chinese believe that each kind of food has its own energy and will have an effect on the body accordingly based on its energy. Therefore, it is important to understand these different energies to improve health.

According to Chinese medicine, great health means a good balance of yin and yang inside of the body. To achieve the state of optimal health, it is recommended you consume foods that can keep your body in balance. The Chinese believe that the human body can be classified into two basic categories: cold types (or yin types) and hot types (or yang types). In other words, it is likely that you tend to have either more yin or yang in the body, which then decides the kinds of foods with the right energies that are required to balance out the excess yin or yang inside your body.

Let me give you a quick definition of what cold and hot body types mean (but I will explain more details in chapter3). If you constantly feel cold and not thirsty and prefer hot or warm drinks, chances are you might have a cold physical constitution (or yin body type) and excess yin. On the other hand, if you tend to feel hot and thirsty all the time and prefer drinking cold drinks, you might have a hot body type (or yang body type) and excess yang.

So far, you've learned the five energies and their benefits to your body. Here's an example of how a certain food can help: if you have a cold body type, it is suggested you consume more ginger, ginseng, and wine, all of which have warm energies that can balance out the excess yin inside the body.

Examples of foods arranged by their different energies are listed in "Appendix A: Foods of Five Energies".

Actions of Foods

There are two types of actions of foods: organic actions and the common actions of foods.

Organic actions of foods refer to specific internal organs on which the foods can act. As you can already tell from "The Five Flavors of Foods", the Chinese focus on ten internal organs for dietary treatments: liver, gall bladder, heart, small intestine, spleen, stomach, lungs, large intestine, kidneys, and bladder. Each food is believed to be able to act on one or more internal organs. And, flavors and energies are important benchmarks to determine the organic actions of foods.

Here are some examples: sweet potatoes act on the stomach; pears act on the lungs; and celeries act on the liver and stomach.

The second type of actions – common actions of foods – refers to the general benefits that foods can bring to you without referring to any specific innate organ. For example, to deal with heat stroke in the summer, you could consider having bitter melons; meanwhile, the same food can also be used for relieving constipation;

23

and, mung beans and Chinese barley are good for reducing breakouts and removing acne marks.

In "Appendix E: Foods of Different Organic and Common Actions", you will find a list of examples for foods with organic actions and common actions.

The Movements of Foods

Before looking into specific directions of these movements, you can first think of the body divided into four regions: inside (internal region), outside (skin and body surface), upper body (above the waist), and lower body (below the waist).

Based on this, TCM has discovered that the energies of foods have a tendency to move inside the body in four directions: upwards, downwards, inwards, and outwards.

To move upwards means to move from lower region to the upper region; foods with upward movements can relieve diarrhea, prolapse the uterus, and promote the falling of the stomach. To move downwards means to move from the upper region to the lower region; so, foods with downward movements may relieve vomiting and hiccupping. To move inwards mean to move from outside to inside; foods with inward movements can ease bowel movements and abdominal swelling. To move outwards mean to move from inside to outside; therefore, foods with outward movements can also induce perspiration and reduce fever – to expel the internal heat out of the body.

As you may have learned already, TCM sees that to heal a certain health issue, you first observe the direction where this particular health issue develops towards; then you use foods with movements of the opposite direction to restore the balance.

To give you a few examples, leaves and flowers tend to move upwards; whereas roots, seeds, and fruits have a tendency to move downwards. But this is only a very general principle; and there are a lot of exceptions.

Besides these four directions, there are also two characteristics associated with food movements: glossy (sliding), and obstructive. Glossy foods (e.g. honey and spinach) can facilitate movements and are good for constipation, and internal dryness. On other hand, obstructive foods (e.g. guava and olive) can prevent movements and are therefore good for diarrhea.

Because of all the healing benefits of foods with different movements, Chinese diets also put a lot of emphasis on this particular food property to select foods accordingly as a way to maintain good health.

Examples of foods arranged by their different movements are listed in Appendix D: "Foods of Four Movements".

By now I hope that you have developed a more intimate relationship with foods and learned to appreciate them through a perspective that's different from the standard approach of using macronutrients (proteins, carbohydrates and fat) and micronutrients (e.g. vitamins and minerals) as the only measures to define nutritional values in foods.

Mother Nature has given you all the signals to appreciate the values from foods. Don't miss out on them.

Next time when you shop for fresh fruits and vegetables at a grocery store, pay attention to their beautiful and juicy colors and think about the associations between these colors and your internal organs.

Similarly, when you sit down for prepared foods at a dining table, don't forget to stay in the moment, enjoy different food flavors, and perhaps show some gratitude for the precious gifts created and sent by the Earth to help you heal and nourish the body from within.

Three Ways to Change Food Energies

Food energies are usually related to foods themselves, in uncooked forms under a normal temperature. But, in reality, we use many ways to store, preserve, and cook foods with different techniques which can lead to changes in food energies. These are the three primary ways that cause food energy changes: the way foods are stored, the way foods are cooked, and the seasonings or ingredients foods are cooked with.

1) The Way Foods Are Stored

In most cases, in order to prolong the shelf life of a certain food, you choose to store it in the fridge or freezer, but this can cool down its energy. For instance, in the summer you might immediately enjoy a cold drink as soon as it is taken out of a cooler or fridge. However, this would bring into the body a lot of cold energies. If you keep doing this on a regular basis, your body will accumulate too much yin energy, which causes imbalances. If you really want to have a cool drink on a hot summer day, wait for a while after the drink is taken out of the cooler or fridge before consuming it. Also, avoid having cold drinks on a regular basis.

2) The Way Foods Are Cooked

Another way to change food energies is to use different cooking methods. Generally, deep drying, toasting, regular frying, stir-frying, boiling, charbroiling, grilling, and steaming foods can all lead to warmer energies in what you eat. You can take advantage of this to cook foods in a way that fits your body type. For example, if you have a yin body type, you can slightly heat up the leafy vegetables – as leafy greens are considered to have yin energies – or prepare a warm veggie soup to balance out the excess yin inside your body.

Not only can you take advantage of cooking methods to restore internal balances, you can also use them to avoid further imbalances as well.

According to TCM, many kinds of animal meat are considered to have warm or hot energies. Can you guess what happens when you charbroil beef, which has warm energies – on a barbecue grill? There will be lots of warm energies accumulated inside the body.

If you consume too much animal meat – whether it is charbroiled, fried, grilled, or stir-fried – in the long run, there will be excess heat accumulated and cause excess yang energy internally. Therefore, one quick tip to avoid excess heat buildup inside the body is to moderate the intake of animal meat prepared with cooking methods that enhance its warm energies.

3) The Seasonings/Ingredients Foods Are Cooked with

The third way to change food energies is to mix in different seasonings or other ingredients. Usually, when you mix scallion, garlic, ginger, chili pepper, or cooking wine with foods, you can easily bring up the energy level. This alters food energies to warm (if the original food energy is cool or cold) or even warmer (if the original food energy is warm or hot).

For example, if you add chopped ginger while cooking eggplants (which have cold energies), this will neutralize the excess cold, making a dish that can serve everybody and suits different body types.

Similarly, when you have hotpot with friends and choose a spicy soup base (which has hot energies), it helps to add in foods with cool energies such as spinach, watercress, and celery to avoid "catching fire" inside the stomach (which means excess heat buildup).

Now it's time for a pop quiz: what happens when you add spices to charbroiled beef on a barbeque grill? Another way to ask this question is: what happens when you add ingredients with *hot* energies to a food (with *warm* energies) cooked in a way that enhances the *warm* energies in foods?

The answer? The final dish will turn out to be having burning hot energies!

As a result, another quick tip is to make sure you only consume beef that has been cooked like this occasionally; and if you have a yang body type, you'd better avoid such meals entirely. Otherwise, you may suffer from excess heat symptoms such as breaking out, dry stool, constipation, and bloating.

Now that you've learned these three ways to alter food energies, you can then wisely and consciously choose to avoid certain dishes cooked in a way that can cause imbalances in your body; and artfully play around with different ways of cooking to come up with the best dishes that fit your body type.

Finally, it is important to remember that there isn't a good or bad way of cooking, only the most suitable way that meets what your body needs.

Six Fundamental Rules to Follow

Below are six tips that encompass the basic principles for healthy eating habits. This is in regard to both what you eat and how you should eat, for the purposes of not only fueling your body, but also nourishing it. These principles are built upon the idea of taking care of the different major organs of your body.

By following these principles, you will discover a restored sense of energy, as well as other benefits, like a new healthy glow on your face.

1) Eat a well-balanced meal.

Basically, having a balanced meal means you should pay attention to these two things: 1) including a wide *variety* of foods into your everyday meals, and 2) knowing how to balance the intake of different foods by giving *priority* to certain types of foods.

First, you should find varieties in food groups, flavors, colors, and different organic actions. That means, you should mix as many types of foods into your diet as possible; such as whole grains, fruits, vegetables, nuts, seeds, and meat (I understand that due to your personal belief or other reasons, you may not consume meat. In that case, make sure you get protein and other essential nutrients from other food groups, like nuts and seeds).

Speaking of vegetables, did you know that different kinds of vegetables have different kinds of energies, too? Generally, yang foods tend to be inward-moving or centripetal; they are usually downward-moving towards the center of the earth. On the contrary, yin foods tend to be more outward-moving split apart or centrifugal; they tend to be upward moving away from the earth. Though it is *not* always true, it is *often* the case. For example, leafy vegetables have cooler energies, whereas root vegetables have warmer energies than leafy ones, in part because they grow under the earth's surface.

In short, you will need to include all leafy, round and root vegetables into your diets to absorb all of their different kinds of energies.

Further, as you continue to eat new varieties of foods, you will also need to include the five flavors (sour, sweet, bitter, pungent, and salty) and colors (green, yellow, red, white, and black) into your everyday meals. Meanwhile, make sure you consciously pick and choose foods that act on different organs to strengthen the body and improve its overall functions.

Second, prioritize certain food groups. As a general rule of thumb, as always, eat whole foods; also, consume more alkaline foods (e.g. dark leafy greens) than acidic foods (e.g. animal proteins); and, prioritize a vegetarian diet with meat only taking up a small portion of your meal, even if you are not a vegetarian or vegan.

Examples of foods arranged by their different food categories and alkalinity are listed in "Appendix G: Foods of Different Alkalinity and Acidity".

2) Design your own balanced diet specific to your own body needs.

As I have already emphasized in my first book – *CHINESE HERBS: Your 101 Guide To Top 10 Chinese Herbs That Clear Up Your Skin And Restore Natural Glow* (http://bit.ly/chinese-herbs), there should not be a generic or standardized nutritional plan for every individual on this planet, because everyone is unique. Therefore, before you go out and ask for what you should eat, you should probably research and find out what kind of body type you have. That's because your special body type decides what you should eat. It is all about supply and demand: because there are demands from your body, you then supply with the right foods it needs to help this piece of machine function better, so that it serves you more efficiently.

So, how do you identify your own body type and what foods you should eat accordingly? I've carved out an entire chapter – Chapter 3 – to discuss this with you, as it's a very important subject.

For now, it is enough to just understand that eating an individualized diet is as important as having a well-balanced diet.

3) Eat till you are 70 – 80 percent full.

Ancient Chinese believe that this ritual is actually very good for your health. That way you are less likely to eat more than your body can digest, or receive more nutrients than your body needs. As a result, you are less likely to gain excess weight, have diabetes, heart diseases, high blood pressure, high blood sugar, or hyperlipidemia.

This practice is also backed up by science as well. When foods enter the stomach, the internal stretch receptors will send a signal to the brain. Yet, this message is not sent instantly – it takes about twenty minutes to arrive at the brain. "You actually feel fuller twenty minutes after you put down your fork", says Dr. Bradley J. Willcox, M.D., a Hawaii-based expert in geriatric medicine and co-investigator of the Okinawa Centenarian Study.

Therefore, if you don't leave the dinner table until you are 100% full. You probably go over the capacity of your stomach at each meal. The worse thing that can happen is that your stomach continues to stretch every time you overeat. Gradually, you will eat more to feel satisfied.

Additionally, according to Dr. Roy Walford – author of *The 12-Year Diet*, proponent of caloric restriction, and participant of the Biosphere 2 project, limiting your daily allowance can prolong a person's life.

4) Eat light meals.

It is beneficial to cut down your fat and sodium intake by reducing the amount of oil and salt you consume. According to Qicheng Zhang, President of the Chinese Medicine Culture Society (which is a branch in_China Association of Traditional Chinese Medicine), it is recommended that one should take no more than 25 grams (about two tablespoons) of oils and no more than six grams of salt per day.

Meanwhile, consume in moderation fried and oily foods; and avoid or cut down the amount of foods with pungent flavors like red chili peppers, scallions and garlics.

Dr. Walford has also made a similar statement. According to him, a low-fat and low-calorie diet rich in nutrients can add more years to your life, and also increase your resistance to diseases in the process.

5) Eat slowly and in a relaxed state.

In today's fast moving society, people tend to eat very fast during their meals. But studies show that eating too fast can easily lead to weight gain. In fact, a previous Japanese study showed that "wolfing down meals could be enough to nearly double your risk of being overweight".

Therefore, it is important to treat yourself to each meal in a tranquil state. Try eliminating all distractions, including television and the internet. Make sure you enjoy and appreciate the food in front of you and the company you are with. It is always a good habit to chew your foods and eat slowly; and take in small bites.

6) Follow the proportions below.

According to my Chinese doctor Fang-Tsuey Lin, fruits and vegetables should make up 50 percent of our everyday food intake. Other than that, 25 percent of your food consumption goes to whole grains, whereas another 25 percent goes to the rest of food groups such as proteins, fats, pickles and miso soup.

To help you better see what to include in your daily diet, here is a pie chart for you:

Whole grains

- Brown rice
- Millet
- Quinoa
- Barley

Others
- Nuts
- Seeds
- Beans
- Pickles
  /sauerkraut
- Miso soup
- Seaweed

Vegetables
- Leafy

- Round

- Root

- Mushrooms
- Fruits

Regarding consuming vegetables, it is important to have different types of vegetables because different types of veggies have different energies. For example, leafy greens have more detoxifying properties and can drive internal energy excesses out of the body, whereas root vegetables are generally more nourishing and have more warm energies.

In addition, TCM sees that it is crucial to introduce more cooked foods into your diets, as they can be more easily digested by the body. On the topic of digestion, you can also start introducing more sauerkraut and miso soup into your daily life as well. They both are good for digestion, which is key to good health and glowing skin.

Tips for You

Another type of seasoning I often use to add saltiness to a dish is miso paste, a traditional Japanese seasoning produced by fermenting soybeans with barley, rice, or other ingredients. This high-sodium food is a good source of protein and dietary fiber and contains three important mineral antioxidants: manganese, copper, and zinc. According to my Chinese doctor, Fang-Tsuey Lin, miso can also effectively protect against radiation poisoning as well.

As for choosing reliable miso, make sure you select certified organic miso to lower your chance of exposure to unwanted contaminants. In addition, my Chinese doctor also suggests choosing miso that is at least two years old. There is one brand that she recommends called South River Organic Miso, which you can find in Whole Foods (if you live in the US). Even if you live outside of the US, you can still stick with the criteria for selecting the best miso possible for your own health.

As you see, in Chinese food therapy there is a standardized guideline that you can follow to have a well-balanced, healthy diet. At the same time, Chinese dietary therapy also takes into consideration that everyone has a unique body; and, therefore, diets should also be individualized. This is the key message that you should take away from this section.

Besides what to eat and how to eat, there is also the important factor of "when" you eat, which is what we are going to discuss next.

How to Eat according to Your Biological Clock

The concept of the Chinese biological clock originated from the two-thousand-year-old *Huangdi Neijing*, or *Yellow Emperor's Inner Canon*, and it is built on the concept of the cyclical ebb and flow of energy throughout the body. During a 24-hour period, the body's energy moves in through two-hour intervals through the 12 meridian systems. This is based upon Traditional Chinese Medicine's belief about pathways through which the life-energy known as "qi" flows.

Each meridian system has its own dominant organ (or a group of organs that perform the same task), which also means that there is one particular organ (or a network of organs) that is most active when qi flows through that particular meridian system at a specific timeframe.

As mentioned in Chapter 1, one thing that makes Chinese food therapy different from other types of diets is its belief in staying in harmony with nature. And one way to respect and follow nature's giving is to understand and eat according to how the body functions internally.

By acknowledging this biological clock designed by nature and understanding how different organs collaborate in 24 hours, you will then better decide when to eat to fit into the body's daily working routine.

For example, if you eat at a time when the stomach is most active, that means foods will be well digested; and if you finish your meal before small intestine is most active, that means the foods you consume are more likely to be turned into nutritional value to fuel the body because small intestine is working hard to absorb the nutrients from foods you take.

The clock inside you shows how different organs inside you are taking turns throughout the 24-hour day as they maintain their functions. This clock tells us when the organs perform at their peak states for different functions such as detoxifying the body, cleansing the blood, digesting foods, and absorbing nutrients.

To make it simple, these are the three time periods ideal for breakfast, lunch and dinner: 7AM – 9AM, 11AM – 1PM, and 5PM – 7PM.

From 7AM to 9AM is when the stomach becomes most active; so, breakfast that you have around this time will be most easily digested. Meanwhile, lunchtime is recommended to be between 11AM and 1PM. This is to make sure that both your breakfast and lunch inside the stomach can catch up with the peak hours that span from 1PM to 3PM, which is when the small intestine is most active, and thus digested most efficiently.

Based on my research, the small intestine is the primary place to digest and absorb proteins; and it takes about three to five hours for the food to pass through the stomach, according to a study conducted by Colorado University. Therefore, I've found out that it is best if you consume more lean protein at breakfast between 7AM and 9AM. That gives your food enough time to pass through the stomach and reach the small intestine for further digestion and for absorption of nutrients (remember, the small intestines are at their peak starting at 1PM).

Dinner time is between 5PM and 7PM. Because the kidneys are considered to be the most active organs at this time, it is recommended to eat less salt, so that you don't dump too much burden on the kidneys. Also, TCM sees that the stomach has the weakest energy from 7PM – 9PM. As a result, it is better to eat light foods that can be easily digested to minimize the workload for the stomach.

The Chinese Biological Clock Explained in Greater Detail

Before we begin, here is something important to consider: you may think that this is too strict of a routine for you, or it is impossible to follow because there are too many "rules". But just know that this is not about being perfect – I found it was very overwhelming to follow everything as soon as I first learned all of this information. This is why it's important to be reminded that this is really about: 1) understanding how your body works for you internally, according to TCM; 2) taking one baby step at a time; and 3) finding what is best for you (or, what fits your lifestyle the most).

I encourage you to get started on this path with the most suitable route you feel comfortable with, while respecting your body's biological clock. In Chapter 4, we will touch more upon getting started into the rhythm of TCM.

Having said that, below is an overview of the Chinese biological clock inside you:

Between 5AM – 7AM: large intestine is most active.

The large intestine is responsible for storing and clearing up waste inside the body. When it is most active, it is recommended you get up early in the morning, and drink enough water to assist bowel movements as well as help with the normal elimination function of the large intestine.

Between 7AM – 9AM: stomach is most active.

When the stomach is at its peak, having breakfast at this time is ideal, as foods are most easily digested when the stomach functions at its best. Another reason for you to enjoy breakfast around this time is that the digested food will then serve nutrients and gives energy to the spleen, which is the next most active organ in the following two hours, to help it better facilitate its jobs.

Besides, as mentioned earlier, it is good to introduce lean protein at this time, so that foods can be digested in time and the nutrients can be more effectively absorbed in a few hours by small intestine when they are most active.

Between 9AM – 11AM: spleen is most active.

After breakfast, the spleen further digests the food you consume early on and starts to collect nutrients from your morning meal; which works to give the spleen more energy to recycle old red blood cells. Chinese Medicine sees that the spleen is connected to your intellectual thinking. That means when the spleen is charged with energy, it is your peak time to conduct work that requires a lot of brain power.

Between 11AM – 1PM: heart is most active.

These are peak hours for movements of qi and blood. Calming down and quieting the mind helps protect the heart at this time. It is highly recommended that you take a nap for at least 10 –15 minutes, but no more than one hour. A Chinese medicine practitioner would tell you that this nap is considered "the golden sleep" to nourish the heart and qi.

Between 1PM – 3PM: small intestine is most active.

During this time, the small intestine is at its peak for digesting foods and absorbing nutrients. It is crucial to make sure you finish your meals before 1PM, so that you can take advantage of the small intestine's function to further break down foods and more effectively extract nutrients from what you eat.

At this time, you could consider drinking more water to bring down excess heat inside the small intestine to restore internal balance, according to TCM.

Between 3PM – 5PM: bladder is most active.

As you may know already, the bladder is an important part of the excretory system to remove excess and unnecessary materials via urination. What you may not know is that this is a time when your brain is very active. So, it is likely that you will increase your productivity if you choose at this time frame to learn something new or review what you've learned.

Similar to what's recommended to take care of your small intestine, drinking water and consuming more fruits around this time can help bring down excess heat inside the bladder.

Between 5PM – 7PM: kidneys are most active.

This is when the kidneys are most active, and it is also the peak time for the kidneys to store energies from all other internal organs. So, it is important to reduce the amount of vigorous exercises. It is also important to moderate the amount of water intake.

And, as mentioned earlier, reduce the amount of salt and eat light for dinner.

Between 7PM – 9PM: pericardium is most active.

The pericardium is a tough double fibrous sac which covers the heart. It protects the heart from infection and provides lubrication. At this time of the day, qi flows through pericardium to nourish the heart and strengthen its functions. It is important to relax yourself and relieve stress at this moment, which can also help with your sleep later on.

Between 9PM – 11PM: Triple Burner is most active.

There is no physical organ associated with Triple Burner system; yet, this was somehow discovered by the ancient Chinese through their observation thousands of years ago. It controls relationships between all organs through the endocrine and hormonal systems. In addition, it is responsible for the movement and transformation of fluids throughout the system, and for the production and circulation of energies.

It is best if you can go to sleep during this time. In fact, this is a major secret for centenarians who live for such a long time. If you choose to not go to bed at this time, you could consider listening to light music, reading for leisure or practicing yoga. And, it is important to keep a balanced and peaceful mind, too.

Between 11PM – 1AM: gallbladder is most active.

This is the most important time of the day, when your body is *crying* for sleep. The body cannot properly facilitate its detoxification and self-renewal process unless you are in deep sleeping mode.

Failing to sleep before 11PM may prevent you from thinking clearly and slow down your thinking process.

Additionally, this is the golden time for renewing skin cells and correcting skin problems It is believed that the better you can follow the routine of sleeping before 11PM, the more likely you are to restore a natural glow from within, plus bright, rosy cheeks. It is that important!

Between 1AM – 3 AM: liver is most active.

Being in deep sleep mode in this time is just as important as sleeping after 11PM. When the liver is most active, it can effectively monitor the contents of the blood and remove many potentially toxic substances before they can reach the rest of the body *when* you are in deep sleep mode. Having said that, you can see that how well the liver functions will directly influence how well the rest of the innate organs function. Not resting well at this period of time can lead to a series of health issues such as blurry vision, palpitation, poor digestion, and rough skin or other skin conditions, just to name a few.

Between 3AM – 5AM: lungs are most active.

Blood goes through lungs to pick up oxygen before returning to the body. How well lungs function determines the quality of the blood the rest of the organs are getting. Again, being in deep sleep mode is crucial to help the body recycle the blood by giving it enough oxygen before distributing it back to the network of organs.

With that said, it is vital to be in sleeping mode between 11PM and 5AM to help your body detoxify and renew itself to start a new day with more energy and a glowing face.

[*Side notes: to learn more about beauty sleep, you could check out my blog here: http://bit.ly/beauty-sleep-benefits.*]

Time-frame	The Most Active Organ (s)	What functions can the Body Perform Best?	Your Recommended Activities Is to....
5AM – 7AM	Large Intestine	Facilitates bowel movements Stores and clear up waste	Wake up Drink water, a lot of water as you get up to stimulate bowel movements
7AM – 9AM	Stomach	Digests foods and absorb nutrients	Enjoy breakfast (preferably with more protein)
9AM – 11AM	Spleen	Digests and absorb nutrients Recycles old red blood cells	Conduct work that requires a lot of thinking
11AM – 1PM	Heart	Peak hours for movement of qi and blood	Take a nap for at least 15 minutes, if possible, but no longer than one hour Have lunch
1PM – 3PM	Small Intestine	Absorbs nutrients Digests foods	Drink water to bring down excess heat inside
3PM – 5PM	Bladder	Removes excess and unnecessary materials via urination Activates your brain	Learn something new or review what you've learned Drink more water Consumer more fruits to help bring down excess heat inside
5PM – 7PM	Kidneys	Store energies from all other internal organs	Reduce the amount of vigorous exercises Moderate the amount of water intake Reduce the amount of salt Eat light for dinner
7PM – 9PM	Pericardium	Protects the heart from infection Provides lubrication	Relax yourself Relieve stress
9PM – 11PM	Triple Burner	Controls relationships between all organs Is responsible for the movement and transformation of fluids throughout the system, and for the production and circulation of energies	Sleep Or, listen to light music, read for leisure, and practice yoga
11PM – 1AM	Gallbladder	Helps the mind stay clear the next day	Sleep
1AM – 3AM	Liver	Monitors the contents of the blood Removes many potentially toxic substances	Sleep
3AM – 5AM	Lungs	Give oxygen to the blood	Sleep

At last, you may be curious about what happens to people who have to travel to another part of the earth and need to deal with time differences. According to my Chinese doctor Fang-Tsuey, your body knows when you reside in a new place and will adjust to local time zone very quickly! But, of course, give your body some time for the adjustment.

45

How to Eat according to Different Seasons

Besides structuring your three meals based on your biological clock, another way that reflects TCM's belief of respecting and following nature is to eat according to different seasons throughout the year.

TCM has discovered that your internal organs are very sensitive to seasonal changes, and that it can be effective in maintaining or improving health if you know how to eat properly to nourish the right organs in the right season. As you already know from "food properties" discussed at the beginning of this chapter, ancient Chinese people understand foods in a slightly different way. They believe that by choosing the right foods with the right flavor, right color, right movement, and right energies in the right season, you can protect and strengthen the body and eventually achieve strong immunity, abundant energy, and that natural glow on your skin.

Before we get started, here is one rule that applies to all seasons; despite the convenience of getting access to foods of all kinds all year-round in the supermarket, it is actually better to give priority to eating foods that are in season. The best way to eat foods in season is to shop at your local farmers markets.

Eating locally grown foods can not only allow you to stay in harmony with nature by taking what it offers you in that particular season, but also ensure you will have the freshest produce with the most nutrients. According to mark Lzeman, Director of Natural Resources Defense Council (NRDC)'s Urban Program in New York, "studies have shown that produce loses nutrients each day after it has been harvested and after three days it has lost 40 percent of its nutritional value". And, shopping locally is healthier for your wallet, too.

Tips for You

If you are currently reside in the US, here is a list of example resources where you can find which foods are in season:

- *Eat Local by Natural Resources Defense Council*
- *Seasonal Food Guide by Sustainable Table*
- *Seasonal Ingredient Map by Epicurious*

Now, in the following section, I will show you the organs you should pay more attention to in different seasons, and the key flavors, movements, energies and colors in foods to look for in each season.

Dietary Advice in Spring

The general tip for eating right in spring is eating foods that are sweet, pungent, with warm energies, liver-nourishing, and with green color. Also, it is important to moderate your intake of sour foods.

Spring is the season of birth and growth. The movements associated with this are outwards (think of an expanding object like a flower blossoming in the spring) and upwards (think of an object growing to a certain height like a young tree becoming taller in the season).

Because Chinese medicine believes that everyone should respect and follow the law of nature, eating proper amounts of pungent foods is one good practice. Foods with pungent flavor can aid perspiration and promote qi movement upwards and outwards, which is in alignment with the movements in spring. Examples of pungent foods include the scallion, onion, garlic, ginger and leek.

In addition to pungent foods, consuming more sweet foods is also crucial in this season to enhance qi, strengthen the functions of the stomach and spleen, and nourish, replenish and tonify other organs. Eating more sweet foods can also keep you in harmony with promoting internal energy flow, too. Examples of sweet foods are honey, sweet fruits, nuts, yams, sweet vegetables like carrots and sweet potatoes, and whole grains like brown rice and millet.

According to TCM, spring dominates liver functioning. And foods with sour taste can tonify the liver. However, you should moderate the intake of sour foods, because consuming too many of them can prevent the spleen from properly functioning. Consuming too many foods with sour flavor may hurt the liver, too. Resulting illnesses can be depression, poor digestion, and menstruation problems. So, watch out for overeating sour foods. Examples are lemon, plum, and grapefruit.

In addition to different flavors of foods, you should also pay attention to the energies of foods you pick. Spring is the right time to start introducing food with warm energies to help nourish the yang energy inside the body. A lot of sweet and pungent foods have warm energies. For more foods with warm energies, you could refer to "Appendix A: Foods of Five Energies".

Because TCM believes that the liver is the organ you should pay the most attention to, nourishing your liver becomes your priority as well. One key way to take care of the liver is to nourish the blood inside the body and to promote blood flow. To do this, you can eat more sesame seeds, goji berries, and Chinese red dates. If you are not a vegan or vegetarian, you could have a small amount of red meat or animal livers. If you become emotional and easily agitated in spring, that means you are likely to have developed excess heat in the liver, which is commonly seen in this season. In that case, sweet foods can help ease your anger or impatience. Other suggestions for food with calming and cooling effects are coconut milk, black sesame seeds, celery, kelp, and watercress.

At last, TCM sees the color green is associated with spring. Therefore, eat more green foods. There is a myriad of benefits resulting from eating more greens; such as cleansing the liver, correcting certain skin problems, improving digestions, and replenishing vitamins, minerals and other nutrients for the body. These are just a few examples of fresh leafy greens to consider: spinach, scallion, lettuce, kale, Swiss chard, turnip greens, and collards. As mentioned earlier, spring is the season with upward movements. And, these leafy veggies have a tendency to move upwards as well – they are planted on earth and grow upwards. That's why consuming more leafy greens is also considered a way to respect and follow laws of nature.

Summary – Dietary Advice in Spring
• *Eat sweet/spleen-nourishing foods*
• *Eat pungent foods*
• *Eat foods with warm energies*
• *Eat liver-nourishing foods*
• *Foods that bring down liver heat*
• *Eat more greens*
• *Moderate intake of sour foods*

Dietary Advice in Summer

In general, summer is the time to take care your heart, lungs, stomach and spleen. Sweet and pungent foods again play a key role, while you need to moderate the intake of foods with bitter flavor (but they can be very helpful in treating symptoms caused by summer heat). It is important to eat light and cut down certain foods with warm or hot energies, like meat and fried foods.

One organ you should pay attention to is the heart. It is easy to develop imbalance in the heart in this hot season manifested as excess heat in the heart, commonly known as "heart fire". If you experience excess heat in summer with symptoms like heat stroke, constipation, skin problems, inflammation, infection, and an aversion to heat, bitter foods are great options for treatment of such imbalances, as this flavor is cooling, descending and contracting. Bitterness can also reduce swelling and encourage bowel movements. Examples of bitter foods are dandelion, chamomile, alfalfa, bitter melon, lettuce, broccoli rabe, and arugula.

Despite the benefits bitter foods can bring, it is important to also moderate the intake of bitter foods in this season, as excess intake of such foods can hurt the lungs, according to TCM. To improve lung functions in the summer, consume more foods with pungent flavors.

Studies show that hot summer weather can cause the nervous system to be in a disrupted state, which leads to poorer digestion and a decrease in appetite. There are two ways to resolve this: on one hand, it is very important to eat light meals by cutting down the intake of meat and fried and oily foods, as they are hard to digest; on the other hand, you can eat more sweet foods to nourish the stomach and spleen to improve appetite.

Summer is also a rainy season. TCM sees that humidity around this time of the year will increase the dampness inside the spleen, which causes other imbalances. In that case, it is important to consume the right foods to drive out the dampness in the spleen. Foods that are good for both nourishing the spleen and getting rid of dampness include: winter melon, pumpkin, ginger, lotus roots, lotus seeds, Chinese barley, and Chinese yam.

Because of the hot summer weather, it is good to balance out the body heat by consuming foods with cooler energies. That also means you should avoid or cut down on foods with hot energies such as fried foods, meat (especially lamb) and lychee. Example foods with cooler energies are water melon, bitter melon, peach, strawberries, tomato, mung bean, and cucumber.

Dietary Advice in Summer
• *Eat sweet/stomach-and-spleen-nourishing foods*
• *Eat pungent/lung-nourishing foods*
• *Eat foods with cooler energies*
• *Foods that can bring down excess heat in heart*
• *Foods that can drive out dampness in spleen*
• *Eat light and cut down meat and fried foods*
• *Moderate intake of bitter foods*

Dietary Advice in Autumn

In this season of dryness, it's best if you have more sweet and sour foods, but reduce the amount of bitter and pungent foods. It's also a good practice to shop for spleen-nourishing and lung-moistening foods. Additionally, the foods you consume should be of neutral or close-to-neutral energies.

In fall, the energy starts to move downwards (think of the falling leaves) and inwards (imagine animals going out, bringing back foods, and storing their foods in their caves to prepare for the coming of winter).

As mentioned earlier, Chinese medicine promotes eating according to the change in nature. And, you've already learned that pungent flavor encourages qi to flow upwards and outwards; which is the reason why it is not recommended to have too many pungent foods in this season. Another reason to reduce the amount of foods with pungency is that they can over strengthen the lungs, which then leads to the weakening of the liver. With the lungs as the dominating organs in fall, TCM thinks it is a good idea to introduce more foods with sour taste into your diet around this time, as they can nourish the liver.

Besides pungency, another flavor to watch out for is bitterness. Too much bitterness in this season can hurt the lungs, according to TCM. This means you may have to cut down the amount of salads, as a lot of raw leafy greens inside salads are bitter tasting, such as lettuce and arugula.

It's not just sourness that can help improve your health at this time. Foods with a sweet flavor can achieve the same result as well.

TCM believes that sweetness can not only nourish the spleen and stomach, but also moisten the lungs. Moistening the lungs is considered the top priority in fall due to the dryness in this season. Consuming more sweet foods can prevent a series of health issues like asthma, upper respiratory infection, dry stool, and skin concerns particularly associated with this season.

Foods that can moisten the lungs include honey, sesame seeds, almond, fruits like apples, bananas, oranges and pears, and vegetables like white radish, carrot, winter melon, white and black fungus, lotus seed, and lily bulb, just to name a few.

Another way to defend dry weather is to make yourself congee in the morning, which is a traditional practice in China proven very effective to nourish the lungs, stomach and spleen, replenish qi, and greatly improve your skin. I've been making congee for breakfast almost every morning these days; and would like to see you join me, too, to enjoy the fun and benefits! In Chapter 6, you will find some of my favorite recipes to help you get started.

Here is one more tip to prevent being caught up by dryness: reduce the amount of foods that can generate internal heat such as lamb, ginger, and fried and oily foods. This is recommended by Ming Li, a Traditional Chinese Medicine practitioner I personal know – based in Newton, Massachusetts – who has been practicing since 1997.

Regarding the energies of the foods that you eat in autumn, it is a good idea to look for foods with more neutral energies. This means it's best to avoid foods with hot or very warm energies like fried and oily foods mentioned above, or foods with very cold energies like raw foods such as salads (which I've already talked about). The recommended foods I bring up above all have neutral or close to neutral energies, and should be consumed on a regular basis in fall.

Dietary Advice in Autumn
• *Eat more sour foods*   • *Eat more sweet/spleen-nourishing foods*   • *Moderate the intake of bitter foods*   • *Moderate the intake of pungent foods*   • *Eat more lung-moistening foods*   • *Eat more foods with neutral or close-to-neutral energies*

Dietary Advice in Winter

In winter, it is most important to nourish the kidneys and heart at the same time. You should have less salty foods and more bitter foods. A general rule of thumb is to eat foods with warm energies while introducing foods with cooler energies from time to time, which can help bring down excess heat inside the body due to the overconsumption of warm foods.

According to TCM, winter is the time to nourish the kidneys. Even though salty foods are considered to be good for the organs, too much salt can hurt the heart. Therefore, the first thing you should do is cut down the intake of salty foods, both to protect the heart and to avoid causing imbalance in the kidneys. At the same time, to prevent the heart from being weakened in the process of nourishing the kidneys, it is important to add more bitterness into your diet.

Due to the cold weather in winter, it then becomes very necessary to introduce more foods with warm energies into your daily life. You need to store enough energy to fight that cold. Example foods with warm energies include lamb, walnuts, chestnuts, cabbage, carrots, red beans, and potatoes. You can also pamper yourself with one small glass of wine to help with blood and qi circulation and to drive out the cold energy.

Additionally, ancient Chinese discovered that the darker the food color goes, the more nutrition it contains, and the more warm energies there are. That's why it is a good idea to introduce more black foods in winter. They will nourish the energy in the kidneys, improve blood circulation, warm up the liver and the rest of the body, and improve functions of the spleen, which TCM believes is a vital organ that keeps other organs working properly. Example black foods are black rice, black bean, black sesame seed, black fungus, and black mushroom.

By now you know that TCM emphasizes a lot on maintaining internal balance, and how having warm foods for the entire winter may cause excess heat, or too much internal yang energy. TCM also reminds you to consume foods with cooler energies from time to time to bring down the heat generated due to overeating of foods with warm energies. You could consider drinking cooled boiled water, or consuming foods with cooler energies such as white radish, lotus seed, cucumber and bitter melon.

Dietary Advice in Winter
• *Eat more bitter/heart-nourishing foods*
• *Eat fewer salty foods*
• *Eat more kidney-nourishing foods*
• *Eat more foods with warm energies*
• *Eat more black foods*
• *Eat foods with cold energies from time to time*

Now I've walked you through all the basics of Chinese Food Therapy. It's like finishing a knitting lesson on basic principles and techniques regarding how to knit. But that's not enough. You will also have to learn how to knit *for yourself* so that you can wear clothes that fit your size. That's what Chapter 3 is about – knowing and discovering your body type, and finding out what's best for YOU.

[Side notes: if you are interested in learning more about seasonal eating, you can check out my book series here - Spring Healthy Guide (http://bit.ly/spring-healthy-eating), Summer Healthy Eating Guide (http://bit.ly/summer-healthy-eating), Autumn Healthy Eating Guide (http://bit.ly/autumn-healthy-eating), Winter Eating Guide (http://bit.ly/winter-healthy-eating), and a collection that combines all of them at a lower price (http://bit.ly/seasonal-healthy-eating).]

Chapter 3: Find Your Body Type and Related Food Solutions

Have you ever noticed that some people may be more easily susceptible to hay fever in spring, while other people seem to be born with a stronger immune system? When you meet new people and shake hands with them in winter, have you ever encountered people whose hands are very cold even when they are wrapped up in warm and thick clothes already, whereas others have much warmer hands to shake with? Are you like me who can easily break out even when I have only a handful of chips, or are you like my husband who doesn't easily have breakouts even after finishing two bags of Frito-Lay?

Different people may react to the same situation differently because each one of us has a different body constitution. TCM sees that body constitution summarizes the individual differences regarding health statuses of organs, qi, blood circulation, mentality and even personality. From a physiological perspective, different body constitutions may reflect individual differences in function, metabolism, and response to external stimuli. From a pathological perspective, it reflects susceptibility of some pathogenic factors, and the tendency for how easily one can develop and transfer certain diseases.

As you learned from Chapter 2, it is not enough to just know a generalized diet plan, because different people have different body constitutions. Different foods may have varied impacts on people with different body constitutions. Understanding your own body type is important, because, with that knowledge, you will be able to customize a diet plan to what your body really needs.

For example, it is recommended to have watermelons and mung beans in the summer to drive out the excess heat inside the body. In the meantime, I have a yin body constitution -- I easily get cold hands and feet in the winter (which I will explain more about later). Therefore, it is better for me to moderate the amount of foods with cold or cool energies such as watermelons and mung beans. Otherwise, I may develop more yin inside the body and become more avoidant of cold in the future. Thus, it is important to first understand if your body has more yin or yang inside of it, to find the right energies in foods that match its needs, and to tweak a standardized meal plan accordingly.

So, what is a yin or yang body constitution? How to find out whether your body type has more yin or yang? This is what we will discover next.

Characteristics of a Yang Body Constitution

In Chinese, the word "yin" means darkness and cold energies; and, the word "yang" means the sun and warm energies. Therefore, generally, a yang body constitution usually describes a body type with more warm energies; and, if you have more yin, this means you might store more yin energies inside your body.

If you have more yang energies inside, it is likely that you have a higher body temperature, are vulnerable to hot weather, and tend to enjoy drinking cold drinks. You may have dry skin.

Personality wise, you may seem to be very energetic, active, outgoing, and able to think, react, and take actions quickly. At the same time, you can easily get impatient, and may be weak at staying disciplined.

With more yang in the body, you may be prone to having dry stool, dizziness, insomnia, palpitation, and a tendency to break out often.

Checklist for Having a Yang Body Constitution

If you have more yang inside the body, it is likely that you...
- *Have a higher body temperature*
- *Are afraid of hot weather*
- *Tend to enjoy cold drinks*
- *May have dry skin*
- *Tend to be energetic, active, outgoing*
- *Are able to think, react, and take actions quickly*
- *Easily get impatient*
- *May be weak at stay disciplined*
- *May be prone to having dry stool, dizziness, insomnia, palpitation, tendency to break out often*

Characteristics of a Yin Body Constitution

Contrary to a person with a yang body constitution, if you have more yin, you tend to have a lower body temperature, are afraid of cold weather, and have the tendency to enjoy hot drinks more.

Personality wise, you are likely to be introverted, and prefer staying in a quiet place with few physical activities. You may oftentimes feel weak and tired, and easily get scared; and it may take you longer time to react to a situation than it takes a person who has more yang.

Typically, a person with a yin body type is prone to having frostbite in the winter, poorer digestion, and swelling.

Checklist for Having a Yin Body Constitution

If you have more yin inside the body, it is likely that you...
- *Have a lower body temperature*
- *Are afraid of cold weather*
- *Have the tendency to enjoy hot drinks more*
- *Are likely to be introverted*
- *Prefer quiet environments*
- *Rarely perform physical activities*
- *Often feel weak and tired*
- *Easily get scared*
- *Respond to a situation more slowly than a person with more yang*
- *May be prone to having frostbite in the winter, poorer digestion, and swelling*

Now that you have a general understanding of both characteristics of yin and yang body constitutions, which do you find applies more to you? If you find yourself fitting into both categories at the same time, it is actually not uncommon at all. As my Chinese doctor, Fang-Tsuey, mentions, it is common to see people in a modern society to have complicated body constitutions. The key is to find out your dominate body constitution -- the one with the more characteristics that apply to you, give priority to it, and take care of your body accordingly.

I am an example of a person with mixed body constitutions. But, I have more characteristics that describe a yin body constitution. Thus, in my daily diets, I will intentionally moderate the amount of foods with cool or cold energies, which will cause a yin body constitution to become more yin.

What happens if you find that neither of the situations apply to you? If that's the case, then it can be good news that you have a more balanced body constitution than most people. With such a constitution, you constantly look energetic, outgoing, positive, and easy-going. And, you find it easy to adapt to external changes, and do not often get sick. It is with this body constitution that one can achieve an optimal state of health and well-being as well as longevity.

Checklist for Having a Balanced Body Constitution

If your internal body is in balance, it is likely that you...
- *Constantly look energized, outgoing, positive, and easy-going*
- *Find it easy to adapt to external changes*
- *Do not easily get sick, or if you do get sick, you can recover very quickly*
- *Look healthy with a natural glow on your face*

Don't worry if you don't have a balanced body constitution yet. Your body is a smart and sophisticated machine that is diligently working to heal itself and restore an internal balance. And, the whole point of adopting Chinese food therapy is to speed up the healing process to help you achieve this balanced body constitution. So, as long as you are following the basic rules by Chinese food therapy, you are moving towards the right direction.

By now, you have learned what yin and yang body constitutions are and which body type(s) you are having. It is time to discuss how to take care of different types of body constitutions.

How to Take Care of a Yang Body Constitution

Chinese food therapy is all about restoring internal balance. Therefore, the general rule is that: if you have more yang in the body, you will need more foods with cool or cold energies. Example foods with cold energies are: bok choy, winter melon, water melon, bitter melon, seaweed, kelp, dandelion, and mulberry. Meanwhile, example foods with cool energies are: corn, pear, banana, celery, cucumber, white radish, taro, mung bean, black fungus, and chrysanthemum.

For more examples of foods with cool and cold energies, visit "Appendix A: Foods of Five Energies" for more references.

How to Take Care of a Yin Body Constitution

If a body with more yang needs to have foods with cool and cold energies, can you guess what energies in foods does a body with more yin needs? The answer is foods with warm and hot energies. It's not hard to guess, is it? Example foods of hot energies are: chili pepper, ginger, and lamb. Example foods with warm energies are: cilantro, pumpkin, scallion, garlic, carrot, bamboo shoot, and fruits like the peach, lychee, organ, and plum.

Again, you can visit "Appendix A: Foods of Five Energies" to check out more foods with warm and hot energies.

How to Take Care of a Balanced Body Constitution

Just because you have a balanced body constitution type, it does not mean that you should stop your efforts. Taking care of the body is just as important for you as for people with more yin or more yang body constitution. Make sure you follow basic principles outlined in Chapter 2 and don't forget to eat more foods in season.

Nine Body Constitutions

Besides understanding your body just from these two big categories -- yin and yang, Prof. Qi Wang, a well-respected professor at the Beijing University of Chinese Medicine, has discovered another way to help you look into your body at a deeper level.

With more than 30 years' hard work in researching body constitutions, he and his team later categorized them into nine different types. Specifically, they are: gentleness, yang deficiency, yin deficiency, qi deficiency, phlegm dampness, dampness heat, blood stasis, qi depression, and special diathesis.

In my book – *CHINESE HERBS: Your 101 Guide To Top 10 Chinese Herbs That Clear Up Your Skin And Restore Natural Glow* – I've covered these nine body types regarding not only dietary advice, but also how to adjust and improve one's lifestyle in general.

We will focus on dietary advice for now, as this book is about dietary therapy. If you want to learn more about these nine body types in more details and how to improve your overall lifestyle to further improve your health and skin, you can find more details from my book at http://bit.ly/chinese-herbs.

Gentleness refers to a well-balanced body type. As mentioned already, a person with a balanced body type will need to continue to embrace a healthy lifestyle and incorporate the basic guidelines from Chapter 2.

As we've already discussed, Yang deficiency refers to an individual who constantly suffers from cold digits no matter what reason it is and is afraid of staying in an air-conditioned environment. If this applies to you, besides consuming more foods with warmer energies, make sure you cut down intake of foods with cold energies like water lemon and cold foods such as ice water and ice cream.

If you constantly feel dehydrated, you probably have a yin deficient body type -- that is, you have more yang in the body. In addition to having more foods with cooler energies, also keep in mind that consuming too many warm or hot foods can bring up internal heat, resulting in more yang and an even more imbalanced body. That's why you need to try to avoid potlucks, pungent and oily foods, lamb, ginger, and lychee.

If you feel that you have poor stamina -- for example, you easily feel tired after you climb only a few stairs, it is likely that you have a qi deficient body constitution. If that's the case, make sure you consume more whole grains like brown rice, oat, and barley, lentils, vegetables, fruits, nuts, and seeds to replenish qi and encourage qi circulation.

Simply put, if you find yourself overweight and not physically fit, then you are likely to have a phlegm dampness body constitution. Eating clean is highly recommended. You can revisit Chapter 2 for more detailed guidelines on getting on a clean diet. In general, consume more fruits and vegetables; and cut down the intake of oily and sweet foods.

Next, if you find that you tend to have acne-prone skin like mine, it is very likely that you have the dampness-heat body constitution. Having a plant-based diet as well as consuming more foods with cooler energies is the key. Two of my favorite foods to combat breakouts, which can also be considered as herbs, are mung bean and Chinese barley. They both have cooling properties. Also, you should especially watch out for warm or hot foods that can bring up your internal heat. Take the example of oily, fried, and pungent foods like red chili peppers, lamb, alcohol, lychee and chips.

Tips for You

Do you know the difference between Chinese barley and other kinds of barley? According to my Chinese doctor, Fang-Tsuey, Chinese barley has more healing benefits and, therefore, can be more effective in producing results. For example, consuming Chinese barley on a regular basis is

> *proven to control breakouts, heal acne marks and brighten up the skin.*

What about blood stasis? A good example to test if you have a blood stasis body type is this: imagine a situation where you accidentally knock yourself over a hard object on a particular part of the body, do you usually get bruises very easily? If you do, do they tend to stay for a long period of time, while having bruises on the skin may not happen to others? If your answers are two yeses, then it's likely that you have a blood stasis body constitution. In this case, it is recommended to consume more foods that aid blood circulation such as fruits like oranges, mandarin oranges, peaches, grapefruits, vegetables like radishes and carrots, herbal teas like green tea and rose tea, marine phytoplankton like algae and seaweed, black beans, etc.

A person with a qi depression body constitution, as you can probably tell from its name, suggests this person often feel depressed and down. If you think this applies to you, try foods that can help qi circulation, relieve depression, improve digestion, and refresh the mind. Examples are whole wheat, cilantro, radish, scallion, mandarin oranges, rose tea, and algae.

The last body constitution is special diathesis. This applies to people with sensitive skin who are prone to allergies. If you think you have this body type, besides having a clean and balanced diet, you will also need to avoid pungent foods like red chili peppers, seafood like shrimps and crabs, drinks like coffee and alcohol, and meat like beef and geese meat.

Here, I would like to remind you again that it is possible if you find yourself fit into more than one category, which is commonly seen nowadays. For example, I have found out that I now have three body constitutions mixed together. The key is to find out what is your dominant body constitution and pay more attention to restoring the imbalances associated, while also taking care of your other imbalances.

To help you efficiently find out your body constitutions and the dominant one, I've simplified the process for you. You can download this excel sheet to find out all the answers in five minutes or less: http://bit.ly/signup-for-bonuses!

Now that you understand what body constitution is, what the different types are, which type(s) of body constitutions you belong to, and the general dietary advice on how to take care of your specific body type(s), the next thing you need to do is integrate what you have just learned into the basic dietary guidelines discussed in Chapter 2. In other words, you need to tweak a common balanced diet a little, so that it becomes more suitable and effective at improving your own health.

Let's go back to the knitting analogy mentioned in the last chapter. Understanding a common dietary guideline is like mastering essential knitting techniques. Identifying your own body type is like measuring your shoulder width, chest width, and waist size. You will need both essential techniques and the right personalized measurements to knit a sweater that perfectly fits you and gives you warmth and protection. Therefore, make sure you combine a common balanced diet with individualized dietary advice based on your own body constitutions.

Now, let's a have a quick overview of what you have learned since Chapter 1.

In Chapter 1, you learned about the brief history and benefits of Chinese food therapy. Then, in Chapter 2, we dove into all the basic principles to follow primarily on guidelines for a common balanced diet. Here, in Chapter 3, we just dug deep to help you discover the importance of getting on a personalized diet and how to customize that diet.

As I always mention in my blog, information without application is useless. So, in the next chapter, I am going to share you my insights on how to get started with Chinese food therapy to help you kick off your journey to more health, naturally glowing skin and longevity.

Chapter 4: Getting Started

This book might have contained a lot of new information to you, and you might be confused about how to get started. This chapter guides you to slowly transition to a Chinese food therapy-inspired lifestyle by holding your hands and taking you one step at a time. I'm about to discuss the overall strategy I suggest, a work plan, specific action steps, and a worksheet you can write on and keep as your "Health Manifesto" which you can revisit from time to time.

In the end – provided that you follow the steps and finish all the fun exercises which come with the chapter – you will come up with a customized diet routine that only serves you, not anyone else. If you are looking for ways to improve your immunity, stay young, healthy, radiant, and feel energetic--there is no better way than nourishing the body from the inside through a personalized plan like this one.

The Strategy

Just like what you need to do to achieve anything in life, the first thing you should consider is not what you can do, but *what results you want to gain*. This helps you stay focused and keep you on track. Therefore, before we dive into the details of how to get into a TCM-inspired diet routine, it is important to take a minute or two to ask yourself what you want to achieve or get from trying out Chinese food therapy. Is your goal to restore glowing and healthy skin, to feel energized, to have good digestion, to improve health, to prevent aging, or to lose weight? (yes, Chinese food therapy can even help you lose weight).

After being clearer about the results you want, the next step is to ask *why you anticipate those results*. This gives you meanings and purposes of switching to a new health habit, and shortens the period of time it takes to transition to this habit. As Tony Robins, the American life coach, self-help author, and motivational speaker, says: a strong enough "why" is the key to pull you through a process of making a change. Thus, to help you stay on course in the process of adapting to Chinese dietary therapy, it is very helpful that you spend another minute or two and ask yourself: "Why do I want to achieve those results I set for myself?" Is your purpose to have a strong body that allows you to purse long-term professional success? Remember that physical health is the foundation for success in anything in life, and you can build confidence by not only looking good, but feeling good, which can lead to the ability to accomplish anything else in life.

At this moment, you are clear about your dream destination and why you want to get there; what follows is *how you can get there*. Before we get started, it is important to know that, throughout the journey, you should also remember to cut down or cut out foods with barely any nutritional value, like white rice, processed foods, refined sugar, artificial sweeteners, canned or microwaved foods, fried foods, packaged pre-bottled fruit, vegetable juices, and packaged foods with additives or artificial ingredients. Make sure you eat whole foods. Additionally, it helps if you can keep a food journal to keep track of what you have been eating, reflect on it, and make adjustments.

Now, let's get to my suggestions to help you transition to a Chinese food therapy-inspired lifestyle.

As Chinese dietary therapy advocates eating to heal the body, you should start from knowing your body first, before choosing what to eat accordingly. Therefore, I recommend you revisit Chapter 3 to understand whether you have more yin or yang inside the body, and take the self-assessment test to find out what body type you have. The goal here is to identity what energies in foods you should prioritize and watch out for.

Next, you are going to keep the knowledge handy and apply it by tweaking a common balanced diet. Doing it is simple. You'll just pay more attention to consuming more foods with the right energies you need and moderating the intake of those with energies that may cause more imbalance. To get started with a common balanced diet, incorporate one new rule into your life every two weeks.

Specifically, in week 1, you can start following the food chart I presented to you in Chapter 2 and introduce more whole grains (preferably in the morning), cooked leafy vegetables, sauerkraut, and miso in your diets.

In week 3, you will start to pay attention to the all flavors of whole foods you consume, identify what they are, and try to make sure you have five flavors – sourness, sweetness, bitterness, pungency, and saltiness – in your everyday meals.

By week 5, you can grow your awareness to the colors of the foods you are eating, and try to incorporate five colors – red, white, yellow, green, and black – into your life (trust me, it is not as hard or complicated as your think).

By the time you begin week 7, you are well on your way to becoming a Chinese food therapy master! This is the time to introduce foods in season. As mentioned in Chapter 2, the best way to enjoy foods in season is to eat locally grown foods. So, in those two weeks, you can explore your local farmers markets for fresh produce to add to your daily meals.

Starting from week 9, you will pay attention to the seasons. Remind yourself of the season you are in at that time and follow the basic principles on seasonal eating laid out in Chapter 2.

It is totally up to you to decide whether you want to use two weeks' time to facilitate a new change in the experiment. As long as you feel comfortable, you could make the interval longer or shorter. The key is to see yourself making progress and allow yourself to try a new diet routine that understands your body, improves its function, and incorporates the laws of nature.

So far, you know what goals you want to achieve, why you want them, and the specific game plan you can utilize to make the shift. I would personally recommend you add one more consideration into your plan – envisioning obstacles.

This means, before you start your first week, you can sit down, pull out a piece of paper, and write down all the possible circumstances that would prevent you from succeeding in following through this plan. According to Kelly McGonical, health psychology professor at Stanford University, installing pessimism in your brain by predicting something unpleasant or unwanted that could happen is twice as likely to help you follow through with a plan compared to giving yourself a lot of positive affirmations. She suggests you adopt both – positive reinforcements and predicting something negative might happen – to ensure you to stick with the plan.

This is why I recommend for you to imagine positive outcomes while visualizing some negative predictions at the same time. To install pessimism and boost your willpower in taking consistent actions, you will need to write down potential obstacles in the middle of the transitioning stage and how you would respond and resolve them.

Work plan*

Preparations: Identify your goals for trying out Chinese food therapy, be clear about why they are important to you, write down potential obstacles you would meet in these 10 weeks** and how you would resolve them, find out your body type and what energies in foods you should prioritize and watch out for, and keep a food journal (optional)

Week 1-2: Incorporate the food chart in Chapter 2

Week 3-4: Make sure you have all flavors - sourness, sweetness, bitterness, pungency, and saltiness – in your daily diet.

Week 5-6: Introduce five colors – red, white, yellow, green, and black – into your meals

Week 7-8: Eat more foods in season and shop more often at local farmers markets

---

Week 9-10: Practice the seasonal eating principles in Chapter 2

*In the entire process, make sure you eat whole foods and cut down or cut out white rice – as it barely has any nutritional value. In addition, processed foods, refined sugar, artificial sweeteners, canned or microwaved foods, fried foods, packaged pre-bottled fruit and vegetable juices, and packaged foods with additives or artificial ingredients should also be disregarded.

**It doesn't have to be 10 weeks. You can prolong or shorten the period, according to your own pace.

To make the transition easier for you, I've simplified the process into eight action steps; each step leads to one statement in the worksheet that follows. You job is to go over each action item, to fill out the worksheet, and to eventually come up with Health Manifesto of your own. You can download a printable worksheet here: http://bit.ly/signup-for-bonuses.

Take Actions Now

Below is a step-by-step guideline for your reference to get started:

- From now on, eat whole foods and cut down or cut out white rice, refined sugar, artificial sweeteners, canned or microwaved foods, fried foods, packaged pre-bottled fruit, vegetable juices, and packaged foods with additives or artificial ingredients

- Write down your health goals you want to achieve after you incorporate Chinese food therapy into your life
- Write down why these goals matter to you
- Review the 10-week plan shown above and write down potential obstacles that can prevent you from proceeding or following through, and how you would respond to them
- Fill out the self-assessment sheet, which can also be found at http://bit.ly/signup-for-bonuses, and go over the checklists in Chapter 3 to find out your body type and whether you have more yin or yang inside the body
- Familiarize yourself with the body constitution you have and recommended dietary advice in Chapter 3
- Follow the 10-week plan
- Take a food journal (optional)

Fill Out the Worksheet/Health Manifesto

From now on, I eat whole foods and cut down or cut out white rice, processed foods, refined sugar, artificial sweeteners, canned or microwaved foods, fried foods, packaged pre-bottled fruit and vegetable juices, and packaged foods with additives or artificial ingredients.

My goal (goals) for trying out Chinese food therapy is (are)   that
_____.
The goal(s) is (are) important to me because
_____
_____.

After reviewing the 10-week plan, I can foresee the following obstacles might happen, but I know how I should handle them.

If by any chance, if you are not so sure of how you should handle the obstacles, you can send me an email and let me help you out! My email is: trcyhuang@gmail.com.

Potential Obstacles	How I Plan to Respond to Them

After revisiting the checklist and taking the self-assessment sheet, I've found out that I have a _____ (yin/yang/mixed/balanced) body constitution.

If the answer above is "mixed", I have also found out that I have more _____ (yin/yang) than _____ (yin/yang), because the checklist for identifying a _____ (yin/yang) body constitution is more applicable to me.

Out of the nine body constitutions, those that apply to me are _____. My dominant body constitution is _____.
Based on the results, I need to have more foods with _____ (hot, warm, neutral, cool, cold) energies; and moderate the intake of foods with _____ (hot, warm, neutral, cool, cold) energies. I know that I can find out foods with different energies in "Appendix A: Foods of Five Energies".

Throughout my 10-week plan, I will remember to add more foods with the energies my body needs and moderate the intake of foods with energies that cause more imbalances in my body.

I follow the 10-week plan and know that I can prolong or shorten the period of time based on my own pace. I know I can turn to the following resources for references:
- Appendix A: Foods of Five Energies
- Appendix B: Foods of Five Flavors
- Appendix C: Foods of Five Colors
- Appendix D: Foods of Four movements
- Appendix E: Foods with Different Organic and Common Actions
- Appendix F: Foods for Nine Body Types
- Appendix G: Foods with Different Alkalinity and Acidity

I can choose to write a food journal to help me reflect on what I eat and make adjustments accordingly.

Are you ready for the journey? Let's turn to the next chapter where I include a 10-week meal plan for you. As you walk through it, you will see that along the way I explain why I design the plan this way and that I share personal tips on how to easily include five flavors and five colors into your everyday meals.

Chapter 5: 10-Week Meal Plan

As mentioned in Chapter 4, each phase is designed to last for two weeks. However, you may choose to progress to the next phase at any time, as long as you feel comfortable in doing so. Once again, throughout the process, make sure you avoid all the bad food choices listed in your Health Manifesto and follow the fundamental rules from Chapter 2 as closely as possible to maximize results.

While you go through these phases, bear in mind your body constitutions, as they will give you a guideline and directions on how you can customize the following suggestions to better fit your body's needs.

Additionally, it is also important to realize that you may not see dramatic changes after only a few weeks. That's because Mother Nature has its own timetable. Your body takes time to adjust to the new lifestyle you bring in; it also takes time for your innate organs to slowly improve their functions and heal themselves. However, slow and gradual changes are more likely to guarantee long-term results. So, the process is well-worth your patience and efforts.

Gradually, you will lose weight, have better digestion, look more energetic, have nourished and brighter skin, and benefit from a body type that's more in balance. As TCM believes that your body constitution is closely connected with your personality, a healthier and balanced body type will naturally lead to a happier and more positive self, too.

Phase 1: Incorporate the food chart in Chapter 2

In this phase, you are about to implement the recommendations laid out in the following chart:
- Vegetables and fruits take up 50 percent of your daily food consumption
- Whole grains, 25 percent
- Other food groups (e.g. proteins and fats) as a whole, 25 percent

Below are basic rules to apply in the first phase:
- You will start to introduce skin-nourishing congee as your breakfast.
- You will gradually incorporate pickles, sauerkraut, and miso paste into your meals.
- Meanwhile, you'll learn to slightly cook the nuts and seeds before consuming them for better digestion.

If you want to drink smoothies, wait until noon or early afternoon when the yang energy is the strongest during the day. It is okay to drink them once or twice in the morning in one week. But, when you consume smoothies first thing in the morning every day, because smoothies contain a lot of cold energies – as they are made of raw foods - drinking them as your breakfast for months or even years may cause too much yin inside the body, which then may cause imbalances and lead to yang deficiency down the road, according to my Chinese doctor Fang-Tsuey.

If, after the self-assessment test, you find out that you have a yang deficiency body type or have more yin inside the body, make sure you follow the rule discussed above when you plan to drink smoothies or other cold energy foods. In addition, it helps to add some slices of ginger inside your smoothies to balance out the energies – as ginger is considered to have warm energies.

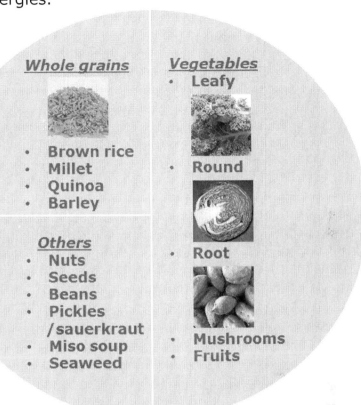

[Check out Phase 1 Sample One-Week Menu here: http://bit.ly/10-week-sample-meal-plan.]

Phase 2: Have all flavors - sourness, sweetness, bitterness, pungency, and saltiness – in your daily diets

At first, I found it a bit overwhelming to keep asking myself after each meal whether I checked off all five flavors. Later, I discovered one quick way to easily incorporate these five flavors into your everyday routine – that is, to build a system, plug yourself into the system, and follow it.

Think about it – if you successfully graduate from Phase 1, this means you are feeling more comfortable with consuming warm water with lemon juice (sour), whole grains (sweet), leafy vegetables (many of which are bitter), sauerkraut (sour), and miso (salty). If you make consuming all the foods mentioned above as a ritual, you have already introduced four flavors into your diets. If the vegetables you consume have no bitter flavor, you can mix turmeric into your meals. What about pungency? Try adding some chopped ginger or slices of ginger in each meal, as consuming a little bit of ginger each day has a myriad of benefits: anti-inflammation, anti-nausea, improving digestion, and helping with absorption and assimilation of nutrients.

As you see, by implementing the getting-started baseline above, you can easily check off five flavors each day. When you have more time and energy, you can then start thinking about bringing in innovative ideas to introduce the five flavors onto your dining table.

[Check out Phase 2 Sample One-Week Menu here: _http://bit.ly/10-week-sample-meal-plan_.]

Phase 3: Introduce five colors – red, white, yellow, green, and black – into your meals.

To add more colors to daily meals, I use the same technique – to create a baseline I can easily follow each day. My personal trick is to add as many colors as possible to my breakfast, the most important meal of the day. That's why you see that very often I add goji berries (red), almonds (white), black sesame seeds (black), fresh herbs like parsley and cilantro (green) into my morning congee made of whole grains like millet, brown rice, and rolled oats (yellow). Occasionally, I pour hemp and flex milk (white) onto my congee to add more lean protein into my diet.

Can you see? You can easily add five colors into one meal! Then, for the rest of the day, I just try to introduce as many colors into my meals as possible without having to worry: "have I added every color into my meals already?"

Of course, you need variety in food choices. But, to just help you kick off Phase 3, it is enough to start with something quick and simple.

[Check out Phase 3 Sample One-Week Menu here: http://bit.ly/10-week-sample-meal-plan.]

Phase 4: Eat more foods in season and shop more often at local farmers markets

I'm so glad that you've made it to Phase 4! You may have noticed already how your skin starts to feel more nourished and moisturized after you consume congee or paste on a daily basis (if you go through each phase for two weeks as suggested). You may have also felt you have better digestion because you regularly consume sauerkraut, miso paste, and the loads of fiber derived from rolled oats and dark leaf greens.

Before we continue, make sure that, as you progress, you incorporate what you learn in previous phases to the existing phase to enjoy full benefits promised by TCM. Therefore, ideally at this time, you have already been able to follow recommendations presented in the food chart and to enjoy foods with five flavors and five colors in your daily meals. Meanwhile, you have also been able customize your diets by incorporating what's good for your body type and by cutting down what's unsuitable for it.

Now, you need to sacrifice a little bit of the convenience of shopping at grocery stores where you can basically buy all kinds of foods regardless of the season. Instead, you will go out to explore your local farmers markets for foods in season. By doing so, you will feel more connected with Mother Nature and eat foods with more nutrients as well.

As we might reside in different places, your area might offer different foods in season than my area. In the following sample one-week menu, I leave this section to your own creativity with what you can buy at your local markets, so that you can start your own experiments with your personal choice.

If you have fun recipes that you would like to share with me, I'd love to receive them all. Just send them over to trcyhuang@gmail.com I look forward to checking out what you create and simply saying hi back to you!

[Check out Phase 4 Sample One-Week Menu here: http://bit.ly/10-week-sample-meal-plan.]

Phase 5: Practice seasonal eating principles in Chapter 2

Congratulations, you've reached the final phase! Have you been reviewing your Health Manifesto from time to time? If yes, that's great. If no, you may want to revisit it to remind yourself of why you are making such efforts in transitioning to Chinese food therapy. This helps you stay on course, keep motivated, and stick with the change, which will definitely benefit you more and more in the long run.

To incorporate seasonal eating principles, you will first have to figure out what season you are in at the moment. Considering you may be reading this book at different times of the year, I have laid out a 8-day menu covering meal plans for different seasons (two days of meal plans for each of the four seasons), so that you can have a sample of what to eat and how to prepare meals in all seasons.

[Check out Phase 5 Sample One-Week Menu here: http://bit.ly/10-week-sample-meal-plan.]

By now, you have been through all five phases. I am sincerely grateful and happy for having you on the journey with me. Let's continue on this path together and stay committed to building vibrant health, which allows you to not only look and feel good, but also build you a strong foundation to help you achieve anything else in life.

This book is a ticket to restoring glowing skin as well as an investment to bring you long-term lifetime value. You may not have realized yet, but you are indeed a smart investor.

Chapter 6: Recipes from Sample Meal Plans

Below are recipes of the dishes mentioned in the last chapter. Names of the dishes are listed in the alphabetical order.

INDEX

A

Astragalus Red Date Shrimp Stew

B

Beef Mixed with Cilantro

Bitter Melon Chrysanthemum Congee

Black Sesame Seeds Congee

Broccoli Rabe with Garlic

Broccoli with Garlic

Brown Rice Sweet Potato Congee

C

Chrysanthemum Lotus Seed Mung Bean Soup

Cilantro Celery Tofu Mix

Creamy Peanut Taro Coconut Soup

F

Fried Eggs with Black Fungus and Onions

Fried Mushrooms with Celeries

Fried Mushrooms and Chinese Cabbage

Fried Mushrooms with Chives and Tofu Skin

G

Ginger Lamb Carrot Soup

Ginger Scallion Garlic Shrimp

Ginger Lettuce Congee with Dates

Green Pepper Tofu Mix

Green Yellow Red White Veggie Garden

H

Home-Made Sauerkraut

K

Kelp Sesame Mix

M

Millet Black Bean Congee

Mixed Veggie Stew

Mung Bean Brown Rice Congee

Mushroom Taro Pumpkin Stew

N

Needle Mushrooms with Fried Eggs

O

Oatmeal Congee with Red Dates

P

Peanut Lotus Root Celery Mix

Peanut White Fungus Congee

Pumpkin Oatmeal Congee

Pumpkin Paste with White Fungus

Purple Cabbage Salad with White Sesame Seeds

S

Seaweed with Egg Soup

Sesame Spinach

Steamed Bass

Steamed Bitter Melon Slices

Steamed Lotus Roots Stuffed with Black Rice

Sweet Sour Yellow-fin Tuna

T

Tomato with Fried Egg

W

Water Chestnut Lotus Root Mix

Whitebait Tofu Stew

White Button Mushrooms with Napa Cabbage

White Radish Mushroom Congee

White Red Green Veggie Mix

Winter Melon Stew

RECIPES

A

Astragalus Red Date Shrimp Stew
Ingredients:
- Shrimps, peeled, 1 cup
- Astragalus, 1/4 cup
- Red dates, 10 pieces
- Ginger, chopped, 2 tbsp
- Clean water, 3 cups
- Himalayan salt, to taste

Serving size:
- 2

Total cooking time (estimated):
- 32 minutes

Preparation time (estimated):
- 2 minutes

Cooking time (estimated):
- 30 minutes

Instructions:
- Add shrimps, astragalus, ginger, and clean water into a pot and bring the water to boil
- Simmer for 20 minutes
- Add red dates into the soup and continue to simmer for 5 minutes
- Turn off heat, add 1-2 pinches of salt, and mix well
- Serve

This dish is especially good for:
- Nourishing the spleen
- Replenishing qi and improving qi circulation
- Warming up the body
- Reducing swelling
- Driving out dampness
- Improving urinary flow
- Treating insomnia

B

Beef Mixed with Cilantro

Ingredients:
- Grass-fed beef, cut into strips, 1 cup
- Cilantro, 4 cups
- Avocado oil, 1 tbsp
- Himalayan salt, to taste

Serving size:
- 2

Total cooking time (estimated):
- 15 minutes

Preparation time (estimated):
- 5 minutes

Cooking time (estimated):
- 10 minutes

Instructions:
- Heat up avocado oil on a frying pan
- Add beef into the pan and sauté with medium to high heat until beef turns from red to brown
- Mix in cilantro and sauté with medium to low heat for 4-5 minutes
- Turn off heat, add 1-2 pinches of salt (add more if needed), and mix well
- Serve

This dish is especially good for:
- Nourishing the spleen and the kidneys
- Giving the body warm energies
- Nourishing qi and blood
- Warming up the body (including the spleen and the stomach)
- Treating shortness of breath

Carrot Cilantro Mix

Ingredients:

- Baby carrots, cut into thin slices, 1 cup
- Ginger, chopped, 1 tbsp
- Cilantro, chopped, 1 cup
- Clean water, 1/3 cup
- Himalayan salt, to taste
- Avocado oil, 1 tbsp

Serving size:
- 1-2

Total cooking time (estimated):
- 15 minutes

Preparation time (estimated):
- 5 minutes

Cooking time (estimated):
- 10 minutes

Instructions:
- Heat up avocado oil on a pan
- Add baby carrots and ginger into the pan and sauté with medium heat for 3-4 minutes
- Add cilantro into the mix and sauté with medium to low heat for 2-3 minutes
- Add 1/3 cup of clean water in the pan and simmer for 2-3 minutes
- Turn off heat, add 1-2 pinches of salt, and mix well
- Serve

This dish is especially good for:
- Lowering down blood lipid levels
- Nourishing qi
- Nourishing the heart
- Preventing heart problems
- Nourishing and brightening up the skin

Bitter Melon Chrysanthemum Congee

Ingredients:
- Bitter melons, cut into small pieces, 1 cup
- Chrysanthemum flowers, 1/3 cup

- Brown rice, 1/2 cup
- Clean water, 4 cups
- (If you want to make savory congee) Himalayan salt, to taste
- (If you want to make the congee sweet) Honey, 2 tsp

Serving size:
- 2

Total cooking time (estimated):
- 53-63 minutes

Preparation time (estimated):
- 3 minutes

Cooking time (estimated):
- 50-60 minutes

Instructions:
- Wash brown rice, add it into water, and bring the water to boil
- Simmer for 40 minutes
- Add bitter melons and chrysanthemum flowers into congee and continue to simmer for another 5 minutes
- Turn off heat
- (If you want to make savory congee) add 1-2 pinches of salt and mix well
- (If you want to make sweet congee) wait until the congee is not burning hot before you add honey and mix well
- Serve

This dish is especially good for:
- Expel summer heat
- Treating heatstroke in summer
- Detoxifying the body
- Brightening up the skin
- Calming the mind

Black Sesame Seeds Congee
Ingredients:
- Rolled oats, 1 cup
- Black sesame seeds, 2 tbsp
- Goji berries, 20 pieces
- Cilantro, chopped, 1/4 cup
- Almonds, 15 pieces
- Clean water, 4 cups
- Himalayan salt, to taste

Serving size:
- 2

Total cooking time (estimated):
- 28 minutes

Preparation time (estimated):
- 3 minutes

Cooking time (estimated):
- 25 minutes

Instructions:
- Add rolled oats, black sesame seeds, almonds, and clean water into a pot and bring the water to boil
- Add goji berries and cilantro into the pot and simmer for 20 minutes
- Add 2 pinches of salt (add more if needed) and mix well
- Serve

This dish is especially good for:
- Nourishing the spleen
- Improving digestion
- Improving vision
- Nourishing the skin and hair

Broccoli Rabe with Garlic
Ingredients:
- Broccoli rabe, 1 bunch
- Garlic, chopped, 2 cloves

- Coconut oil, 1 tbsp
- Avocado oil, 1 tsp
- Himalayan salt, to taste

Serving size:
- 2

Total cooking time (estimated):
- 14 minutes

Preparation time (estimated):
- 5 minutes

Cooking time (estimated):
- 9 minutes

Instructions:
- Cut off and discard the tough ends of the broccoli rabe, cut the rest into 2-inch pieces, rinse them under running water, and drain them
- Heat up the pan with avocado oil with medium to high heat
- Add garlic into the pan and cook until garlic turns brown
- Lower the heat to medium to low, add pieces of broccoli rabe into the pan, and sauté for 4-5 minutes
- Add 1-2 pinches of salt into the pan, mix well, and continue to sauté for another 1-2 minutes
- Turn off heat, add coconut oil, and mix well
- Serve

This dish is especially good for:
- Detoxifying the liver
- Improving digestion
- Preventing cancer
- Slowing down aging process

Broccoli with Garlic

Ingredients:
- Broccoli, 1 head broccoli
- Garlic, chopped, 5 cloves

- Ginger, chopped, 2 tbsp
- Avocado oil, 2 tbsp
- Himalayan salt, to taste
- Clean water, 1/2 cup (for cooking the broccoli stem)
- Clean water, 1/2 cup (for cooking the florets added later on)

Serving size:
- 2-3

Total cooking time (estimated):
- 10 minutes

Preparation time (estimated):
- 5 minutes

Cooking time (estimated):
- 5 minutes

Instructions:
- Trim off the florets, cut off the "trunk" of each floret to make bite-sized pieces, and place florets in a bowl (Bowl A)
- Trim and slice the stem and place the pieces in a separate bowl (Bowl B)
- Heat up the frying pan with avocado oil with medium to high heat
- Add chopped garlic and ginger into the pan and stir fry until garlic starts to turn brownish
- Lower the heat to medium to low, add in ingredients in Bowl B and 1/4 cup of clean water, cover up the pan with a lid, and cook for 1 – 1.5 minute
- Add in ingredients in Bowl A and 1/4 cup of clean water, cover up the pan again, and cook for 1.5 - 2 minutes
- Remove the lid, add in one or two pinches of salt, and mix well
- Serve

This dish is especially good for:

- Improving your immune system because studies show that broccoli has antibacterial and antioxidant properties and because garlic alone also has antibacterial properties as well

Note:

This is a good example that shows how a simple and easy-to-make dish can contain loads of nutritional benefits to help you become stronger and healthier. As soon as you remove the lid, you will immediately be attracted by the smell of this dish. Additionally, it not only smells good, but tastes very good as well.

Pumpkin Millet Congee

Ingredients:
- Millet, 1 cup
- Pumpkin, peeled and cut into bitable chunks, 4 cups
- Clean water, 7 cups

Serving size:
- 4

Total cooking time (estimated):
- 50 minutes

Preparation time (estimated):
- 5 minutes

Cooking time (estimated):
- 45 minutes (actual cooking is just about 10 minutes)

Instructions:
- Wash millet, add it to water 3 cups of water, and bring the water to boil
- Simmer for 25 minutes
- (While cooking millet), add pumpkin chunks and 4 cups of water into a blender, blend the mixture into a paste, and pour the paste into a bowl for later use

- (After simmering for 25 minutes) add pumpkin paste into the congee, stir well, and continue to simmer for another 15 minutes
- Turn off heat and serve

This dish is especially good for:
- Nourishing the skin
- Improving digestion
- Fighting wrinkles
- Lowering blood sugar level
- Preventing cancer
- Calming the mind

Brown Rice Sweet Potato Congee

Ingredients:
- Sweet potatoes, peeled and chopped into bitable pieces, 1 cup
- Brown rice, 1/3 cup
- Ginger, chopped, 2 tbsp
- Cilantro, cut into small pieces, 1/2 cup
- Coconut oil, 1 tbsp
- Clean water, 3 cups

Serving size:
- 1-2

Total cooking time (estimated):
- 50 minutes

Preparation time (estimated):
- 5 minutes

Cooking time (estimated):
- 45 minutes

Instructions:
- Wash brown rice, place brown rice and sweet potatoes into the water, and bring the water to boil
- Add in ginger and simmer for 40 minutes
- Turn off heat, add in cilantro and coconut oil, and mix well

- Serve

This dish is especially good for:
- Nourishing the spleen and the stomach
- Improving digestion
- Improving bowel movements
- Protecting joints
- Nourishing the respiratory system

Notes:

I personally add cilantro and coconut oil into the congee because they both contain antioxidant properties, which help you improve your immunity. Additionally, they both add refreshing and pleasant flavors to the dish, too.

C

Chrysanthemum Lotus Seed Mung Bean Soup

Ingredients:
- Chrysanthemum flowers, 1/2 cup
- Lotus seeds, with embryos removed, 1/4 cup
- Mung beans, 1/2 cup
- Clean water, 4 cups

Serving size:
- 2

Total cooking time (estimated):
- 56 minutes

Preparation time (estimated):
- 1 minute

Cooking time (estimated):
- 55 minutes

Instructions:
- Place lotus seeds and mung beans into water and bring the water to boil
- Simmer for 45 minutes
- Wash chrysanthemum flowers, place them into the soup, and continue to simmer for 5 minutes

- Turn off heat and serve

This dish is especially good for:
- Clearing excess heat in the heart and the body
- Brightening up the skin
- Potentially removing dark spots
- Calming the mind
- Replenishing and nourishing qi
- Preventing cancer
- Lowering blood pressure
- Driving out dampness
- Healing acne breakouts
- Improving immunity

Cilantro Celery Tofu Mix

Ingredients:
- Celeries, sliced, 1 cup
- Tofu, cut into small bitable chunks, 1 cup
- Cilantro, 1 cup
- Dried black fungus, 1/3 cup
- Himalayan salt, to taste
- Sesame oil, 2 tsp
- Avocado oil, 2tbsp
- Clean water, 2 cups (for soaking black fungus)

Serving size:
- 2

Total cooking time (estimated):
- 18 (plus 4 hours for soaking black fungus)

Preparation time (estimated):
- 5 minutes (plus 4 hours for soaking black fungus)

Cooking time (estimated):
- 13 minutes

Instructions:
- Soak black fungus for 4 hours
- Rinse black fungus under running water and darin fungus

- Add 2 tbsp of avocado oil on a frying pan and heat up the oil
- Add tofu chunks into the pan and sauté with medium heat till they become golden
- Add black fungus into the pan and sauté for 2-3 minutes
- Mix in celery slices and cilantro and sauté with medium to low heat for 3-4 minutes
- Turn off heat, add 2 pinches of salt and sesame oil, and mix well
- Serve

This dish is especially good for:
- Enriching the blood
- Nourishing the stomach, the kidneys, and the heart
- Preventing heart problems
- Detoxifying the body
- Improving digestion

Creamy Peanut Taro Coconut Soup

Ingredients:
- Raw peanuts, 1/2 cup
- Taro, peeled and cut into small bitable chunks, 1 cup
- Organic coconut cream, 2 tbsp
- Clean water, 1 cup (for soaking peanuts for 4 hours)
- Clean water, 4 cups

Serving size:
- 2

Total cooking time (estimated):
- 60 minutes

Preparation time (estimated):
- 5 minutes

Cooking time (estimated):
- 55 minutes (plus 4 hours for soaking peanuts)

Instructions:
- Soak peanuts for 4 hours
- Add peanuts and 2 cups water into a pot and bring the water to boil
- Simmer for 30 minutes
- Add taro chunks and 2 cups of water into the same pot and again bring the water to boil
- Simmer for 15 minutes
- Add coconut cream into the pot, mix well, and continue to simmer for 1-2 minutes
- Turn off heat and serve

This dish is especially good for:
- Nourishing and moisturizing the skin
- Improving brain functions
- Slowing down aging process
- Strengthening heart functions
- Reducing phlegm
- Relieving coughs
- Nourishing yin energy
- Nourishing qi
- Nourishing the lungs, the stomach, the spleen, and the heart

F

Fried Eggs with Black Fungus and Onions
Ingredients:
- Black fungus, 1/3 cup
- Onions, chopped into small pieces, 1 cup
- Organic eggs, 4
- Avocado oil, 2 tbsp
- Himalayan salt, to taste

Serving size:
- 2-3

Total cooking time (estimated):
- 16 minutes plus 4 hours for soaking black fungus

Preparation time (estimated):
- 5 minutes plus 4 hours for soaking black fungus

Cooking time (estimated):
- 11 minutes

Instructions:
- Soak black fungus for 4 hours
- Rinse black fungus under running water and drain fungus
- Break eggs into a bowl, stir well, and make them into a paste
- Add 1 tbsp of avocado oil into a frying pan and heat up the pan
- Lower the heat to medium to low, pour egg paste into the pan, and sauté for 1-2 minutes until egg paste becomes solid
- Use turner to cut cooked egg paste into pieces and place cooked egg pieces into a container
- Add 1 tbsp of avocado oil into a frying pan and heat up the pan
- Lower the heat to medium, add black fungus into the pan, and sauté for 2-3 minutes
- Add chopped onions into the pan and sauté onions and fungus for 2-3 minutes
- Add egg pieces and 2-3 pinches of salt into the pan and continue to sauté for 1-2 minutes
- Turn off heat and serve

This dish is especially good for:
- Improving immunity
- Nourishing the kidneys, the stomach, the spleen, and the lungs
- Enriching the blood and qi
- Lowering blood lipid level
- Prevent heart diseases
- Detoxifying the body
- Prevent cancer
- Slowing down aging process

Fried Mushrooms with Celeries

Ingredients:
- Dried mushrooms, 1/2 cup
- Celeries, chopped into small chunks, 10 stalks
- Himalayan salt, to taste
- Avocado oil, 2 tbsp
- Sesame oil, 1 tsp

Serving size:
- 3

Total cooking time (estimated):
- 11 minutes + 1 night for soaking the dried mushrooms

Preparation time (estimated):
- 5 minutes + 1 night for soaking the dried mushrooms

Cooking time (estimated):
- 6 minutes

Instructions:
- Soak dried mushrooms in water overnight (about 6 to 10 hours)
- Wash the mushrooms in running water, rinse them, and drain them
- Cut mushrooms into thin slices
- Heat the pan with medium to high heat and add avocado oil
- When your hand can feel the heat by hovering over the oil, add in slices of mushrooms and chopped celeries, stir fry with medium heat for about 5 minutes
- Sprinkle one to two pinches of salt and mix well (add more if need be)
- Turn off heat, wait till the dish cools down a little, add sesame oil and mix well
- Serve

This dish is especially good for:

- Driving heat in the liver to bring this organ back to balance
- Relieving high blood pressure, heart diseases, and hyperlipidemia
- Improving immune system
- Fighting cancer
- Fight radiation
- Slowing down aging process
- Nourishing the skin, the liver, the kidneys, the stomach, and the spleen
- Improving qi and blood flow in the body

Fried Mushrooms and Chinese Cabbage

Ingredients:
- Dried mushrooms, 8 pieces
- Chinese cabbage, sliced, 4 cups
- Ginger, minced, 1 tsp
- Scallion, chopped into small pieces, 1/3 cup
- Clean water, enough to soak 8 pieces of mushrooms
- Avocado oil, 1 tbsp
- Sesame oil, 1 tsp
- Himalayan salt, to taste

Serving size:
- 2

Total cooking time (estimated):
- 25 minutes (plus 6-8 hours for soaking the dried mushrooms)

Preparation time (estimated):
- 10 minutes (plus 6-8 hours for soaking the dried mushrooms)

Cooking time (estimated):
- 15 minutes

Instructions:
- Wash mushrooms till they are clean

- Soak mushrooms overnight (about 6-8 hours, the amount of water just enough to cover the mushrooms)
- Remove the stems, cut mushrooms into slices, and place them aside (save the water used to soak mushrooms)
- Add avocado oil into the pan and heat the oil with medium heat
- Add in ginger and slices of mushrooms and sauté for 5 minutes
- Add in sliced cabbage and sauté with medium to low heat for 3 minutes
- Pour the water used to soak mushrooms into the pot and continue to cook for 3-4 minutes (with lid on top of the pot)
- Add 2 pinches of salt, chopped scallions, and sesame oil into the pot and mix well (add more salt if needed)
- Turn off heat and serve

This dish is especially good for:
- Replenishing qi and improving qi circulation inside the body
- Lowering blood lipid levels
- Lowering blood sugar levels
- Improving immunity

Fried Mushrooms with Chives and Tofu Skin
Ingredients:
- Dried mushrooms, 6 pieces
- Bamboo shoots, cut into 2-inch strips, 1 cup
- Chives, cut into 2-inch pieces, 2 cups
- Tofu skin, sliced into thin strips, 2cups
- Avocado oil, 2 tbsp
- Himalayan salt, to taste
- Clean water, 2 cups

Serving size:

- 2-3

Total cooking time (estimated):
- 25 minutes (plus 6-8 hours for soaking dried mushrooms)

Preparation time (estimated):
- 10 minutes (plus 6-8 hours for soaking dried mushrooms)

Cooking time (estimated):
- 15 minutes

Instructions:
- Wash and soak dried mushrooms in 2 cups of clean water overnight for 6-8 hours
- Rinse soaked mushrooms under running water and drain them
- Cut mushrooms into thin slices
- Heat up avocado oil in a frying pan with medium to high heat
- Lower the heat to medium and add mushrooms slices and bamboo shoots into the pan and sauté for 5 minutes
- Add tofu skin strips into the mix and continue to sauté for 3-4 minutes
- Add chives into the pan and sauté with medium to low heat for 2-3 minutes
- Turn off heat, add 2-3 pinches of salt into the pan, and mix well
- Serve

This dish is especially good for:
- Boosting the mood
- Losing weight
- Nourishing the kidneys and the stomach
- Enriching qi and blood

G

Ginger Lamb Carrot Soup
Ingredients:

- Ginger, sliced, 15g
- Lamb, 250g
- Baby carrots, 1 cup
- Cooking wine, 1/4 cup
- Clean water, 2 cups
- Clean water, 2 cups
- Himalayan salt, to taste

Serving size:
- 2

Total cooking time (estimated):
- 190 minutes

Preparation time (estimated):
- 7 minutes

Cooking time (estimated):
- 180 minutes

Instructions:
- Bring 2 cups of clean water to boil, add lamb into the boiling water, cook it for 30 seconds, and run lamb under tap water for about 10-15 seconds
- Put ginger, lamb, carrots, and 2 cups of clean water into a pot and bring the water to boil
- Add cooking wine into the mixture and simmer for about 3 hours (with the lid on the top of the pot)
- Add one or two pinches of salt (add more if needed)
- Serve

Ginger Scallion Garlic Shrimp

Ingredients:
- Shrimps, peeled, 1 cup
- Ginger, chopped, 3 tbsp
- Apple cider vinegar, 1 tbsp
- Organic soy sauce, 1 tbsp
- Garlic, chopped, 3-4 cloves

- Scallions, 1/4 cup
- Sesame oil, 2 tsp
- Clean water, 2 cups
- Avocado oil, 2 tbsp

Serving size:
- 2-3

Total cooking time (estimated):
- 15 minutes

Preparation time (estimated):
- 5 minutes

Cooking time (estimated):
- 10 minutes

Instructions:
- Bring the water to boil
- Add shrimps into boiling water and boil shrimps until they become red
- Drain shrimps and place them on a plate
- Heat up avocado oil on a frying pan with medium to high heat
- Lower the heat to medium, add ginger and garlic, and sauté until garlic turns brown-ish
- Lower the heat to medium to low, add apple cider vinegar, soy sauce, and scallions and mix well
- Turn off heat, add sesame oil, and mix well
- Pour sauce evenly onto shrimps
- Serve

This dish is especially good for:
- Detoxifying the body
- Warming up the body
- Slowing down aging process
- Fighting colds
- Nourishing the spleen, the stomach, and the lungs
- Relieving coughs
- Relieving diarrhea

Ginger Lettuce Congee with Dates

Ingredients:
- Ginger, chopped, 2 tbsp
- Lettuce, chopped, 3 cups
- Brown rice, 1/3 cup
- Red dates, pitted and cut into pieces, 8 pieces
- Clean water, 2 cups

Serving size:
- 2

Total cooking time (estimated):
- 45 minutes

Preparation time (estimated):
- 5 minutes

Cooking time (estimated):
- 40 minutes

Instructions:
- Add brown rice, ginger, and red dates into a pot, mix them with water, and bring the water to boil
- Simmer for another 35 minutes (with the lid on the top of the pot)
- Add lettuce into the pot and continue to simmer for 5 minutes (with the lid on top of the pot)
- Serve

This dish is especially good for:
- Nourishing the stomach, the spleen, the heart, and the lungs
- Expelling the coldness out of the body and keeping the body warm
- Treating digestive issues that cause nausea, vomiting and diarrhea
- People who suffer from hyperglycemia and heart diseases
- Preventing you from cancer
- Treating health issues related with the respiratory system such as asthma and phlegm in the lungs

Notes:

Traditionally, ginger and red dates have been used together for deep healing benefits. You could also try mixing both to make yourself Chinese herbal tea to gain similar benefits mentioned above.

Green Pepper Tofu Mix

Ingredients:
- Dried tofu, chopped into small bitable pieces, 1 cup
- Green peppers, with seeds removed and sliced, 2 cups
- Cilantro, chopped, 1/4 cup
- Clean water, 4 cups
- Sesame oil, 2 tsp
- Himalayan salt, to taste

Serving size:
- 2-3

Total cooking time (estimated):
- 15 minutes

Preparation time (estimated):
- 5 minute

Cooking time (estimated):
- 10 minutes

Instructions:
- Bring the water to boil
- Place tofu chunks into boiling water, cook for 1-2 minutes, and drain tofu chunks
- Place green pepper slices into boiling water, cook for 1 minute, and drain green pepper slices
- Place tofu chunks and green pepper slices into a bowl, add in 1-2 pinches of salt, sesame oil, and cilantro, and mix well
- Serve

This dish is especially good for:
- Nourishing qi

- Moisturizing the body
- Expelling internal heat
- Detoxifying the body
- Improving digestion
- Improving appetite

Green Yellow Red White Veggie Garden
Ingredients:
- Peas, 1/2 cup
- Corns, 1/2 cup
- Baby carrots, cut into small bitable pieces, 1/2 cup
- Potatoes, peeled and cut into small bitable chunks, 1/2 up
- Cucumbers, cut into small bitable chunks, 1/2 cup
- Ginger, chopped, 3 tbsp
- Scallions, chopped, 1/4 cup
- Avocado oil, 3 tbsp
- Himalayan salt, to taste
- Clean water, 2 cups

Serving size:
- 3-4

Total cooking time (estimated):
- 30 minutes

Preparation time (estimated):
- 15 minutes

Cooking time (estimated):
- 15 minutes

Instructions:
- Add 2 cups of water into a pot and bring the water to boil
- Add carrot pieces and potato chunks into boiling water and cook for 3 minutes
- Turn off heat and drain carrot pieces and potato chunks

- Heat up avocado oil on a frying pan with medium to high heat
- Lower the heat to medium, add ginger and scallions into the pan, and sauté for 1 minutes
- Add carrot pieces, potato chunks, peas, corns, and cucumber chunks into the pan and continue to sauté for 3-4 minutes
- Turn off heat and add 3 pinches of salt (add more if needed)
- Serve

This dish is especially good for:
- Nourishing the skin
- Improving digestion
- Strengthening stomach functions
- Relieving coughs
- Improving immunity
- Preventing cancer
- Preventing heart diseases
- Nourishing qi

H

Home-Made Sauerkraut

Ingredients:
- Cabbage, enough to fill one 25-ounce Mason jars
- Ginger, chopped, 1 tbsp
- Clean water, 1/3 cup

Total cooking time (estimated):
- 12 minutes (disregarding the time it needs for fermentation)

Preparation time (estimated):
- 2 minutes

Cooking time (estimated):
- 10 minutes (disregarding the time it needs for fermentation)

Instructions:

- Keep 2-3 outer leaves of the cabbage for later use
- Add 1 tbsp of chopped ginger into the Mason jar
- Peel off layers of cabbage, cut them into small pieces, pack the jar with pieces of cabbage as tight as possible, but leave out 1-inch space between the top of the jar and the cabbage
- Add water into the jar
- Roll up 2 cabbage leaves, and pack them on the top of the pieces of cabbage
- Cover the jar with a lid and make sure the jar is air-tight
- Leave the jar at a dark, cool, and dry place for 3-5 days
- When it's done (check out "notes" below to see how to tell when it is ready to be served), twist off the lid and discard the two rolls of cabbage leaves
- Place the jar in the fridge to keep it fresh

This dish is especially good for:
- Improving digestion
- Nourishing the skin
- Promoting overall health due to its amount of vitamins, minerals, and enzymes

Notes:
- Fun fact: I actually learned about making sauerkraut from nutritionist Kimberly Snyder in her book *The Beauty Detox Solutions:* *http://bit.ly/beauty-detox-solutions.* ;)
- You can make this throughout the year and consume it regularly. Depending on which season you prepare sauerkraut, the time it takes for making the sauerkraut varies. According to my experience, it takes about 2-3 days in summer and about 4-5 days in winter before the sauerkraut is ready to be served. Usually, the time when you can tell it's done is when you see

the size of pieces of cabbage start to shrink, leaving extra space inside the jar.
- When the sauerkraut is ready, it is normal to see air bubbles starting to appear and hear sizzling sounds as you twist off the lid. So, don't have to freak out.

K

Kelp Sesame Mix
Ingredients:
- Kelp, cut into 2-inch strips, 1 cup
- White sesame seeds, 2 tbsp
- Sesame oil, 2 tsp
- Organic soy sauce, 1-2 tsp
- Clean water, 2 cups

Serving size:
- 2

Total cooking time (estimated):
- 25 minutes

Preparation time (estimated):
- 3 minutes

Cooking time (estimated):
- 22 minutes

Instructions:
- Bring 2 cups of water to boil
- (While boiling water) heat up a frying pan with medium to high heat
- (While boiling water) lower the heat to medium, add sesame seeds into the pan, sauté until you can smell white sesame seeds and they start to turn brown-ish
- (While boiling water) turn off heat and place sesame seeds in a bowl for later use
- (When the water is boiled) add kelp strips into boiling water and cook for 15 minutes
- Drain kelp strips and place them in a bowl

- Mix kelp strips and white sesame seeds together
- Add soy sauce and sesame oil into the same bowl and mix well
- Serve

This dish is especially good for:
- Nourishing hair and skin
- Detoxifying the body
- Reducing swelling
- Driving out excess heat inside the body
- Preventing heart diseases

M

Millet Black Bean Congee

Ingredients:
- Millet, 1/4 cup
- Black beans, 1/4 cup
- Goji berries, 30 pieces
- Clean water, 4 cups
- Cilantro, chopped, 1/2 cup

Serving size:
- 2

Total cooking time (estimated):
- 57 minutes

Preparation time (estimated):
- 2 minutes

Cooking time (estimated):
- 55 minutes

Instructions:
- Mix millet, black beans, goji berries, and clean water into a pot and bring the water to boil
- Add in goji berries and simmer for 50 minutes (with a lid on the top of the pot)
- Turn off heat, add cilantro into the pot, and mix well
- Serve

This dish is especially good for:

- Improving your immune system because of the benefits from nutrient-dense millet, which is especially good for those who have a weak body type
- Nourishing the liver, the spleen and the kidneys
- Improving vision
- Treating anemia and constipation
- Women's reproductive system

Mixed Veggie Stew
Ingredients:
- Corns, 1/2 cup
- Winter melons, peeled and cut into small chunks, 1 cup
- Chinese yam, peeled and sliced, 1/2 cup
- Broccoli, cut into small florets, 2 cups
- Dried mushrooms, 10 pieces
- Lettuces, chopped into small pieces, 2 cups
- Baby carrots, sliced, 1 cup
- Clean water, 5 cups
- Clean water, 1 cup (for soaking dried mushrooms)
- Miso paste, 2 tbsp
- Avocado oil, 1 tbsp
- Sesame oil, 1 tbsp

Serving size:
- 5

Total cooking time (estimated):
- 58 minutes (plus 6-8 hours for soaking dried mushrooms)

Preparation time (estimated):
- 15 minutes (plus 6-8 hours for soaking dried mushrooms)

Cooking time (estimated):
- 43 minutes

Instructions:

- Wash dried mushrooms and soak them in 1 cup of clean water overnight for 6-8 hours
- Keep the water and cut soaked mushrooms into thin slices
- Add corns, winter melon chunks, Chinese yam, mushrooms slices, baby carrot slices, 5 cups of water, and 1 cup of water used for soaking dried mushrooms into a pot and bring the water to boil
- Add avocado oil into the pot, mix well, and stew with medium heat for 30 minutes
- Add miso paste into the stew and mix well
- Add broccoli florets and lettuce into the stew, mix well, and stew with medium to low heat for 2-3 minutes
- Turn off heat, add sesame oil, and mix well
- Serve

This dish is especially good for:
- Improving immunity
- Improving appetite
- Strengthening stomach functions
- Improving digestion
- Relieving coughs
- Bringing down internal heat and excess dampness
- Preventing heart diseases and cancer
- Reducing swelling

Mung Bean Brown Rice Congee

Ingredients:
- Mung beans, 1/2 cup
- Brown rice, 1 cup
- Clean water, 4 cups

Serving size:
- 4

Total cooking time (estimated):

- 46 minutes

Preparation time (estimated):
- 1 minute

Cooking time (estimated):
- 45 minutes

Instructions:
- Wash mung beans and brown rice, add them into clean water, and bring the water to boil
- Simmer for 40 minutes (with lid on top of the pot)
- Turn off heat and serve

This dish is especially good for:
- Detoxifying the body
- Relieving thirst
- Reducing swelling
- Driving out internal heat
- Calming the mind

Mushroom Taro Pumpkin Stew

Ingredients:
- Pumpkin, peeled and cut into small bitable chunks, 2 cups
- Taro, peeled and cut into small bitable chunks, 2 cups
- Dried mushrooms, 12
- Scallions, chopped, 1/4 cup
- Coconut cream, 1/4 cup
- Avocado oil, 2 tbsp
- Himalayan salt, to taste
- Clean water, 1 cup (for soaking dried mushrooms)
- Clean water, 6 cups

Serving size:
- 4

Total cooking time (estimated):

- 37 minutes (plus 6-8 hours for soaking dried mushrooms)

Preparation time (estimated):
- 10 minutes (plus 6-8 hours for soaking dried mushrooms)

Cooking time (estimated):
- 27 minutes

Instructions:
- Wash mushrooms and soak them overnight for 6-8 hours
- Heat up avocado oil on a frying pan, lower the heat to medium, add in scallions, and sauté till you can smell scallions
- Add pumpkin chunks and taro chunks into the pan and fry till they are brown-ish
- Pour everything inside the frying pan into a pot and add mushrooms, water used for soaking mushrooms, and 6 cups of clean water into the same pot
- Bring the water to boil
- Simmer for 15 minutes or until pumpkin chunks and taro chunks become soft
- Add in coconut cream, mix well, and continue to simmer for 2 minutes
- Turn off heat and add 3-4 pinches of salt (add more salt if needed)
- Serve

This dish is especially good for:
- Improving digestion
- Lowering down blood sugar levels
- Nourishing and brightening up the skin
- Preventing cancer
- Detoxifying the body

N

Needle Mushrooms with Fried Eggs

Ingredients:
- Needle mushrooms, 2 cups,
- Organic eggs, 2
- Avocado oil, 2 tbsp
- Himalayan salt, to taste

Serving size:
- 2

Total cooking time (estimated):
- 11 minutes

Preparation time (estimated):
- 1 minute

Cooking time (estimated):
- 10 minutes

Instructions:
- Break 2 eggs into a bowl, stir them into an egg paste
- Cut off and discard the bottom of needle mushrooms
- Rinse the mushrooms under running water and drain them
- Add avocado oil on a frying pan, add mushrooms into the pan, and sauté with medium heat for 3-4 minutes
- Pour egg paste onto needle mushrooms, wait for about 30 seconds, and sauté mushrooms every few seconds until egg paste is fully cooked
- Turn off heat, add 1-2 pinches of salt, and mix well
- Serve

Oatmeal Congee with Red Dates

Ingredients:
- Rolled oats, 1/2 cup
- Chinese red dates, pitted, 6 pieces

121

- Clean water, 2 cups
- Raisins, 2 tsp
- Himalayan salt, to taste

Serving size:
- 1-2

Total cooking time (estimated):
- 22 minutes

Preparation time (estimated):
- 2 minutes

Cooking time (estimated):
- 20 minutes

Instructions:
- Add rolled oats into water and bring the mixture to boil (with the lid on top of the pot)
- Add in Chinese red dates and simmer for 15 minutes
- Turn off heat
- Add in 1-2 pinches of salt (add more if needed) and raisins
- serve

This dish is especially good for:
- Improving digestion
- Preventing heart problems
- Nourishing the skin
- Enriching and replenishing
- Bringing down blood pressure

Notes:
- If you are allergic to gluten like me, try gluten-free rolled oats.

P

Peanut Lotus Root Celery Mix

Ingredients:
- Raw peanuts, 1 cup
- Celeries, chopped into small bitable chunks, 1 cup

- Lotus roots, peeled and chopped into small chunks, 1 cup
- Tea bags with jasmine tea, 2
- Clean water, 2 cups (for soaking peanuts)
- Clean water, 3 cups (for cooking peanuts)
- Clean water, 1 cup (for cooking lotus roots and celeries)
- Sesame oil, 1 tbsp
- Cilantro, chopped into small pieces, 1/2 cup
- Himalayan salt, to taste

Serving size:
- 4

Total cooking time (estimated):
- 115 minutes plus 4 hours for soaking peanuts

Preparation time (estimated):
- 5 minutes plus 4 hours for soaking peanuts

Cooking time (estimated):
- 110 minutes

Instructions:
- Soak peanuts in clean water for 4 hours
- Drain peanuts and place soaked peanuts, 2 jasmine tea bags, 3 cups of water into a pot
- Bring the water to boil and simmer for 30 minutes
- Turn off heat, pour the water, peanuts, and teabags into a contains, and let the mixture sit for another 60 minutes
- Add 1 cup of clean water into a frying pan and bring the water to boil
- Lower the heat to medium high, add lotus and celery chunks, and sauté for 5 – 10 minutes
- Drain lotus root and celery chunks and place them in a bowl
- Drain peanuts and mix nuts into lotus root and celery chunks
- Add cilantro, 3-4 pinches of salt, and sesame oil and mix well

- Serve

This dish is especially good for:
- Nourishing the stomach and the spleen
- Nourishing the lungs
- Relieving phlegm
- Replenishing qi
- Moistening the throat
- Fighting aging
- Improving memory
- Nourishing the skin
- Reducing swelling

Peanut White Fungus Congee

Ingredients:
- Raw peanuts, 1/2 cup
- Brown rice, 1/2 cup
- Dried white fungus, 1
- Clean water, 5 cups
- Honey, 1 tbsp

Serving size:
- 4

Total cooking time (estimated):
- 60 minutes (plus 2 hours for soaking white fungus)

Preparation time (estimated):
- 5 minutes (plus 2 hours for soaking white fungus)

Cooking time (estimated):
- 55 minutes

Instructions:
- Soak white fungus for 2 hours or till it is soft
- Cut white fungus into small pieces and rinse them under running water
- Wash brown rice, put peanut, pieces of white fungus, and brown rice into water in a pot, and bring the water to boil

- Simmer for 50 minutes (with lid on top of the pot)
- Turn off heat, add honey into the mix, and stir well
- Serve

This dish is especially good for:
- Moisturizing the skin
- Anti-aging
- Improving memory
- Improving brain functions
- Treating heart diseases and high blood pressure
- Improving qi circulation
- Nourishing the spleen, the stomach, and the lungs

Pumpkin Oatmeal Congee

Ingredients:
- Rolled oats, 1/2 cup
- Brown rice, 1/2 cup
- Pumpkin, peeled, pitted, and chopped into small bitable chunks, 4 cups
- Clean water, 6 cups
- Scallions, chopped, 1/4 cup
- Himalayan salt, to taste

Serving size:
- 4

Total cooking time (estimated):
- 65 minutes

Preparation time (estimated):
- 5 minute

Cooking time (estimated):
- 60 minutes

Instructions:
- Wash brown rice, add brown rice and 4 cups of water into a pot, and bring the water to boil
- Simmer for 30 minutes

- (While simmering) Add pumpkin chunks and 2 cups of water into a blender and blend them into a pumpkin paste
- (After simmering brown rice for 30 minutes) pour pumpkin paste into the congee and continue to simmer for 10 minutes
- Add rolled oats into pumpkin congee and continue to simmer for 15 minutes
- Turn off heat, add in scallions and 3-4 pinches of salt, and mix well
- Serve

This dish is especially good for:
- Replenishing and nourishing qi
- Detoxifying the body
- Improving immunity
- Nourishing and moisturizing the skin
- Improving digestion
- Calming the mind

Pumpkin Paste with White Fungus

Ingredients:
- Pumpkin, peeled, pitted, and chopped into small bitable chunks, 2 cups
- White fungus, 1
- Red dates, pitted, 6-8 pieces
- Goji berries, 20 pieces
- Honey, 1 tbsp (optional)
- Clean water, 2 cups (for soaking white fungus)
- Clean water, 3 cups

Serving size:
- 2-3

Total cooking time (estimated):
- 45 minutes (plus 3-4 hours for soaking white fungus)

Preparation time (estimated):
- 5 minutes

Cooking time (estimated):
- 40 minutes (plus 3-4 hours for soaking white fungus)

Instructions:
- Soak white fungus in 2 cups of water for 3-4 hours
- Rinse white fungus under running water, cut it into small pieces, and place pieces of white fungus in a pot
- Add 2 cups of water into the pot
- Bring the water to boil
- Add plus red dates and goji berries into the pot, mix well, and simmer for 30 minutes
- (While simmering) add 1 cup of water and pumpkin chunks into a pan and bring the water to boil
- (While simmering) simmer pumpkin chunks for 10-15 minutes
- (While simmering) pour pumpkin chunks and water inside the pot into a blender and blend away
- (While simmering) pour pumpkin paste into a bowl for later use
- (After simmering white fungus for 30 minutes) pour pumpkin paste into white fungus soup and mix well
- Turn off heat
- (Optional) add honey and mix well
- Serve

This dish is especially good for:
- Nourishing the spleen and the stomach
- Improving appetite
- Nourishing qi
- Calming the mind
- Treating insomnia
- Nourishing yin
- Expelling heat out of the body

- Nourishing the lungs
- Moisturizing the skin

Purple Cabbage Salad with White Sesame Seeds
Ingredients:
- Purple cabbage, sliced, 2 cups
- Scallions, chopped, 1/4 cup
- Sesame oil, 2 tsp
- Cilantro, cut into small pieces, 1/3 cup
- White sesame seeds, 1-2 tbsp
- Red chili oil, to taste (optional)
- Himalayan salt, to taste

Serving size:
- 2

Total cooking time (estimated):
- 5 minutes

Preparation time (estimated):
- 2 minutes

Cooking time (estimated):
- 3 minutes

Instructions:
- Wash and drain white sesame seeds and cook them on a pan with medium to low heat until they are dry and become brown-ish
- Mix slices of purple cabbage, scallions, sesame oil, cooked white sesame seeds, and cilantro together into a bowl
- Add 2 pinches of salt into the mixture (add more if needed)
- Add 1-2 tsp of red chili oil into the mixture (add more if needed)
- Stir well and serve

This dish is especially good for:
- Nourishing the skin
- Treating various kinds of skin issues such as itchiness and eczema

- Anti-aging
- Losing weight
- Improving immunity
- Preventing you from catching a cold
- Relieving joint pains
- Bringing down inflammation
- Improving digestion and alleviate constipation

Notes:
- If you have sensitive and acne-prone skin like mine, then red chili oil is not recommended. As TCM believes that red chili oil can bring up internal heat inside your body which already has excess heat (if you have acne-prone skin). Therefore, consuming red chili oil may lead to breakouts.

S

Seaweed with Egg Soup

Ingredients:
- Roasted seaweed, 15 g
- Organic egg, 1
- Clean water, 2 cups
- Himalayan salt, to taste

Serving size:
- 1

Total cooking time (estimated):
- 9 minutes

Preparation time (estimated):
- 1 minutes

Cooking time (estimated):
- 8 minutes

Instructions:
- Bring the water to boil
- Turn the heat down to medium to low heat, add in roasted seaweed, and stir well until seaweed

becomes soft (the process should be only about 2 minutes)
- Turn off heat, break the egg into the pot, stir well in circular motion until the egg is cooked
- Add in 1 pinch of salt

Serve
- This dish is especially good for:
- Nourishing the heart and body
- Expel summer heat
- Preventing heart problems and high blood pressure (if you consume seaweed on a regular basis)
- Improving immunity
- Preventing you from cancer
- Improving memory
- Improving urinary flow
- Removing phlegm

Notes:
- I suggest only 1 pinch of salt because seaweed already tastes a little salty. As a result, you actually don't need that much sodium into your soup.

Sesame Spinach

Ingredients:
- Baby spinach, 8 cups
- White sesame seeds, 2 tbsp
- Clean water, 4 cups
- Himalayan salt, to taste
- Sesame oil, 2 tsp

Serving size:
- 2

Total cooking time (estimated):
- 10 minutes

Preparation time (estimated):
- 1 minutes

Cooking time (estimated):
- 9 minutes

Instructions:
- Heat up white sesame seeds on the pan and sauté until sesame seeds turn brown-ish
- Turn of heat, place sesame seeds on a plate, and set the plate aside for later use
- Bring the water to boil, place spinach into the pot, lower the heat to medium to low, and cook till spinach becomes soft
- Drain spinach and place spinach on a plate
- Mix in white sesame seeds, 1-2 pinches of salt, and sesame oil and stir well
- Serve

This dish is especially good for:
- Improving digestion
- Improving immunity
- Improving metabolism
- Slowing down aging process
- Moisturizing the body
- Nourishing yin energy inside the body
- Enriching and replenishing blood
- Calming the mind
- Bringing down internal heat

Steamed Bass

Ingredients:
- Bass, sliced, 2 cups
- Scallions, chopped, 1/4 cup
- Ginger, 2 tbsp
- Garlic, chopped, 2 cloves
- Organic soy sauce, 1 tbsp
- Apple cider vinegar, 1 tbsp
- Avocado oil, 2 tbsp
- Goji berries, 10 pieces
- Sesame oil, 2 tsp

- Clean water, 2 cups

Serving size:
- 2

Total cooking time (estimated):
- 25 minutes

Preparation time (estimated):
- 10 minutes

Cooking time (estimated):
- 15 minutes

Instructions:
- Add 2 cups of clean water into the bottom of a steamer and bring it to boil
- (While boiling water) mix fish fillets with goji berries and 1 tbsp of avocado oil and place them on a plate
- (When the water is boiled) place the plate with fish fillets into the rack of the steamer and steam with medium to high heat for 6 minutes
- Take fish fillets out of the steamer
- Heat up a frying pan with 1 tbsp f avocado oil with medium to high heat
- Lower the heat to medium, add ginger and garlic into the pan, and sauté until garlic turns brownish
- Lower the heat to medium to low, add scallions, organic soy sauce, and apple cider vinegar into the pan, and sauté for 1-2 minutes
- Turn off heat, add sesame oil, mix well with the sauce in the frying pan, and quickly pour sauce evenly on the fish fillets
- Serve

This dish is especially good for:
- Treating anemia
- Nourishing the liver, the spleen, and the kidneys
- Strengthening spleen functions
- Nourishing qi
- Improving digestion

- Warming up the body

Steamed Bitter Melon Slices

Ingredients:
- Bitter melons, with seeds removed and cut it into thin slices, 2 cups
- Clean water, 4 cups
- Himalayan salt, to taste
- Sesame oil, 4 tsp

Serving size:
- 4

Total cooking time (estimated):
- 15 minutes

Preparation time (estimated):
- 5 minutes

Cooking time (estimated):
- 10 minutes

Instructions:
- Place water at the bottom of the steamer and bring it to boil
- Place bitter melon slices onto the rack and make sure slices are evenly spread out
- Steam for 3-5 minutes
- Take bitter melon slices out into a bowl
- Mix with 1- 2 pinches of salt and sesame oil and stir well
- Serve

This dish is especially good for:
- Bringing down internal heat
- Driving out dampness
- Activating skin cells and brightening the skin
- Improving vision
- Cleansing your liver
- Detoxifying your body
- Treating acne breakouts
- Bringing down blood sugar level

-   Losing weight
Notes:
-   You could add more salt if you want. But make
    sure you don't add too much. The point of
    adding salt here is to just slightly enhance the
    flavor. Too much salt can make the dish tastes
    too heavy and too much of saltiness does not
    blend well with bitterness. And, it is not good for
    your health either by making the dish too salty.

Steamed Lotus Roots Stuffed with Black Rice

Ingredients:
-   Lotus root, peeled, 1 (about 6 inches long)
-   Black rice, 1/2 cup
-   Honey, 1 tbsp
-   Clean water, 4 cups (for boiling the lotus root)

Serving size:
-   2

Total cooking time (estimated):
-   39 minutes (disregarding the time needed to
    cool down the stuffed lotus roots and to cut it
    into thin slices)

Preparation time (estimated):
-   1 minutes plus 3-4 hours for soaking black rice

Cooking time (estimated):
-   38 minutes (disregarding the time needed to
    cool down the stuffed lotus roots and to cut it
    into thin slices)

Instructions:
-   Wash black rice and soak it for 3-4 hours
-   Cut off one end of the lotus root
-   Stuff soaked black rice into the holes
-   Place the piece of lotus root that has been cut
    off back to its original spot to seal the holes and
    prevent black rice from dropping out (you can
    use 2 or 3 toothpicks to hold two parts together

– the part that has been cut off and the rest of the lotus root)
- Put 4 cups of water into a pot and bring it to boil
- Place stuffed lotus into the pot and steam with medium heat for 30 minutes
- Turn off heat, take stuffed lotus root out of the pot, and let it sit until the temperature cools down
- Cut the stuffed lotus root into thin slices (an image is attached below for your reference)
- Dip slices of stuffed lotus root into honey and serve

This dish is especially good for:
- Nourishing and moistening the lungs
- Clearing summer heat
- Nourishing the spleen and the stomach
- Treating diarrhea
- Reducing agitation due to hot weathers
- Improving blood circulation
- Improving appetite
- Enriching, replenishing, and nourishing the blood
- Fighting free radicals
- Improving immunity

Sweet Sour Yellow-fin Tuna

Ingredients:
- Yellow-fin tuna fillets, 17 ounce
- Green peppers, chopped into bitable pieces, 1/3 cup
- Avocado oil, 2 tbsp
- Honey, 1 tbsp
- Vinegar, 1 tbsp
- Cooking wine, 2 tbsp
- Ginger, chopped into small pieces, 2 tbsp
- Scallions, chopped into small pieces, 1/4 cup
- Clean water, 1/2 cup

- Himalayan salt, to taste

Serving size:
- 2

Total cooking time (estimated):
- 17 minutes

Preparation time (estimated):
- 5 minutes

Cooking time (estimated):
- 12 minutes

Instructions:
- Heat up the frying pan with avocado oil
- Place tuna fillets on the pan and fry with medium to high heat for 2 minutes
- Flip the fish fillets over and cook the other side with medium to high heat again for 2 minutes
- Add 1/2 cup of water into the pan, lower the heat to medium, and stew for 4-5 minutes
- Place the fish fillets onto a plate and set aside
- Place green pepper pieces into the same frying pan and sauté with medium to low heat for 1-2 minutes
- Turn the heat to medium to low, add in scallion pieces, ginger pieces, vinegar, honey, cooking wine, and 2 pinches of salt, and mix well
- Turn off heat and spread the seasoning evenly onto the fillets
- Serve

This dish is especially good for:
- Anti-aging
- Preventing cancer
- Fighting free radicals
- People with anemia
- Replenishing qi
- Improving qi flow
- Treating insomnia

T

Tomato with Fried Egg

Ingredients:
- Tomatoes, cut into small pieces, 6
- Organic eggs, 4
- Garlic, chopped, 2 cloves
- Celery stalks, chopped into small pieces, 2
- Himalayan salt, to taste
- Clean water, 1 cup
- Avocado oil, 2 tbsp
- Sesame oil, 2 tsp

Serving size:
- 3

Total cooking time (estimated):
- 20 minutes

Preparation time (estimated):
- 5 minutes

Cooking time (estimated):
- 15 minutes

Instructions:
- Crack the eggs into a bowl, mix them up until a yellow paste is formed, set the bowl aside for later use
- Heat the pan with 1 tbsp of avocado oil using medium to high heat
- Add in the egg paste, turn the heat to medium to low, and let it sit without stirring until the bottom of the egg paste becomes solid and forms a thin slice of an egg pancake
- Turn the egg pancake over with the turner and cook the other side for about 15-30 seconds (it doesn't matter if you break the cooked egg paste into pieces, because you are going to break the pancake into small pieces later on anyway)

- Use the edge of the turner to cut the cooked egg pancake into small bitable pieces right in the frying pan
- Place egg pancake pieces into a bowl and set the pieces aside for later use
- Add 1 tbsp of avocado oil into the pan and heat it up with medium to high heat
- Lower the heat to medium, add in garlic and cook until garlic starts to turn brown-ish and you can smell it
- Add in tomato pieces and sauté for 2-3 minutes
- Add 1 cup of water into tomato pieces and stew with medium to low heat for 5 minutes
- Use the turner to press the tomato pieces so that tomato juices come out into the soup
- Add egg pancake pieces and chopped celeries into tomato soup and stew with medium to low heat for 2-3 minutes (this step help egg pancake pieces absorb as many tomato juice as possible)
- Turn off heat and add in 2-3 pinches of salt and sesame oil
- Serve

This dish is especially good for:
- Improving immunity
- Nourishing the skin
- Lowering blood pressure
- Strengthening the stomach
- Improving appetite and digestion
- Driving out internal heat
- Detoxifying the body
- Nourishing the liver
- Preventing heart problems

W

Water Chestnut Lotus Root Mix
Ingredients:

- Water chestnuts, peeled and cut into bitable pieces, 1 cup
- Lotus roots, cleaned, peeled, and cut into bitable pieces, 1 cup
- Clean water, 2 cups
- Himalayan salt, to taste

Serving size:
- 2-3

Total cooking time (estimated):
- 35 minutes

Preparation time (estimated):
- 10 minutes

Cooking time (estimated):
- 25 minutes

Instructions:
- Bring the water to boil
- Add in water chestnut and lotus root pieces and simmer for 20 minutes
- Turn off heat, add 1-2 pinches of salt, and mix well
- Serve

This dish is especially good for:
- Nourishing the spleen and the stomach
- Expelling heat and dampness
- Treating diarrhea

Whitebait Tofu Stew

Ingredients:
- Dried whitebaits, 1/2 cup
- Fresh tofu, cut into small pieces, 2 cups
- Clean water, 3 cups
- Cooking wine, 2 tbsp
- Ginger, sliced, 3-4 pieces
- Sesame oil, 2 tsp
- Himalayan salt, to taste

Serving size:

- 2

Total cooking time (estimated):
- 18 minutes plus 30-60 minutes for soaking dried whitebaits

Preparation time (estimated):
- 3 minutes plus 30-60 minutes for soaking dried whitebaits

Cooking time (estimated):
- 15 minutes

Instructions:
- Soak dried whitebaits for 30 – 60 minutes
- Bring the water to boil
- (While boiling the water) wash tofu pieces and whitebaits
- Add tofu, whitebaits, ginger slices, and cooking wine into boiling water and stew for 10 minutes with medium heat
- Turn off heat, add sesame oil and 1-2 pinches of salt, and mix well
- Serve

This dish is especially good for:
- Nourishing yin energy
- Nourishing the stomach
- Replenishing qi
- Relieving coughs

White Button Mushrooms with Napa Cabbage

Ingredients:
- Napa cabbage, cut into 2-inch strips, 4 cups
- White button mushrooms, cut into thin slices, 1 cup
- Avocado oil, 1 tbsp
- Sesame oil, 1 tsp
- Himalayan salt, to taste
- Black pepper, to taste
- Clean water, 1/3 cup (to cook napa cabbage)

Serving size:
- 2

Total cooking time (estimated):
- 18 minutes

Preparation time (estimated):
- 10 minutes

Cooking time (estimated):
- 8 minutes

Instructions:
- Add oil to pot and heat oil with medium to high heat
- Turn the heat to medium, add in strips of napa cabbage to pot and 1/3 cup of water, and cook till cabbage become soft and about 70% cooked
- Add in slices of mushrooms and sauté until mushrooms are cooked
- Turn off heat, add 1-2 pinches of salt, 1-2 pinches of grinded black pepper, and sesame oil into the pot, and mix well
- Serve

This dish is especially good for:
- Nourishing the stomach
- Lowering the lipid levels in the blood
- People with heart disease and high blood pressure

White Radish Mushroom Congee

Ingredients:
- White radishes, peeled and cut into small bitable chunks, 2 cups
- Dried mushrooms, 10 pieces
- Brown rice, 1 cup
- Ginger, sliced, 3-4 slices
- Goji berries, 30 pieces
- Cilantro, chopped into small pieces, 1/2 cup
- Sesame oil, 3 tsp

- Clean water, 5 cups
- Himalayan salt, to taste

Serving size:
- 3

Total cooking time (estimated):
- 55 minutes plus 6-8 hours for soaking mushrooms

Preparation time (estimated):
- 5 minutes plus 6-8 hours for soaking mushrooms

Cooking time (estimated):
- 50 minutes

Instructions:
- Wash mushrooms and soak them overnight in 2 cups of water (about 6-8 hours)
- Add mushrooms along with water used for soaking mushrooms, chunks of white radishes, brown rice, and another 3 cups of water into a pot
- Bring the water to boil
- Add slices of ginger and goji berries into the pot and simmer for 45 minutes
- Turn off heat, add 2-3 pinches of salt, sesame oil, and cilantro into the soup, and mix well
- Serve

This dish is especially good for:
- Improving immunity
- Nourishing and moistening the lungs
- Detoxifying the body
- Relieving constipation
- Improving urinary flow
- Improving digestion
- Reducing phlegm

White Red Green Veggie Mix
Ingredients:

- Potatoes, peeled and cut into 2-inch strips, 1 cup
- Baby carrots, sliced, 1 cup
- Green bell peppers, with seeds removed and sliced, 1 cup
- Scallions, chopped, 1/4 cup
- Apple cider vinegar, 1-2 tbsps
- Avocado oil, 2 tbsp
- Himalayan salt, to taste
- Sesame oil, 2 tsp

Serving size:
- 2

Total cooking time (estimated):
- 29 minutes

Preparation time (estimated):
- 15 minutes

Cooking time (estimated):
- 14 minutes

Instructions:
- Heat up a frying pan with avocado oil
- Lower the heat to medium, add scallions into the pan, and sauté for 30-40 seconds
- Add potatoes strips into the pan and sauté for 3-4 minutes
- Add sliced carrots into the pan and continue to sauté for 3-4 minutes
- Lower the heat to medium to low, add apple cider vinegar and 2 pinches of salt, mix well, and continue to sauté for 1-2 minutes
- Add green pepper slices into the pan and continue to sauté for 1-2 minutes
- Turn off heat, add sesame seed oil, and mix well
- Serve

This dish is especially good for:
- Nourishing the spleen and the stomach
- Driving out dampness
- Bringing down inflammation

- Detoxifying the body
- Improving digestion
- Bringing down blood sugar levels
- Nourishing qi and blood
- Reducing swelling
- Improving immunity
- Slowing down aging process
- Relieving constipation
- Improving stamina
- Relieving joint pains
- Treating eczema

Winter Melon Stew

Ingredients:
- Winter melons, peeled and chopped into bitable chunks, 1 cup
- Dried mushrooms, 8 pieces
- Ginger, chopped into small pieces, 2 tbsp
- Scallions, chopped into small pieces, 1/4 cup
- Clean water, 1 cup (for soaking dried mushrooms)
- Clean water, 1 cup
- Sesame oil, 2 tsp
- Himalayan salt, to taste

Serving size:
- 2

Total cooking time (estimated):
- 22 minutes

Preparation time (estimated):
- 5 minutes plus 6-8 hours for soaking dried mushrooms overnight

Cooking time (estimated):
- 17 minutes

Instructions:

- Wash dried mushrooms and soak fried mushrooms overnight (about 6-8 hours) in 1 cup of water
- Cut mushrooms into small pieces
- Place pieces of mushrooms, water used to soak mushrooms overnight, winter melon chunks, and 1 more cup of water into a pot
- Bring the water to boil and simmer for 10 minutes
- Add ginger, scallions, and 2 pinches of salt into the stew and continue to simmer for another 2 minutes
- Turns off heat, add in sesame oil, and mix well
- Serve

This dish is especially good for:
- Bringing down summer heat
- Improving immunity
- Driving out dampness
- Weight loss
- Nourishing the lungs
- Reducing swelling
- Stimulate bowel movements
- Preventing cancer
- Lowering blood sugar level

Check Out My Other Books

Congratulations on finishing this book! I hope you have already started trying out some of the recipes listed for you and are having fun with making new dishes.

These dishes are taken out from my seasonal eating book series. If you are interested in learning how to keep your body healthy in different seasons and how to take care of the skin by consuming the right foods in the right way in the right season, then I highly recommend you check out my book series on seasonal eating.

Each book I wrote contains more than 60 recipes to help you get started and gives you tips on how you can alter the way you eat slightly differently in different seasons to promote longevity, restore health and beauty, and constantly cultivate peace in the mind (yes, good foods nourish not only the body but the mind as well).

Let me know how you like the dishes and perhaps send me a few pictures of what you have made (again, here's my email: trcyhuang@gmail.com). I'd love to hear from you and learn from your thoughts and insights in this journey.

Below is a list of my books on seasonal eating:

Healthy Eating: Spring Healthy Eating Guide and 60+ Recipes Inspired by Traditional Chinese Medicine to Detoxify the Body and Achieve Optimal Health: http://bit.ly/spring-healthy-eating.

Healthy Eating: Summer Healthy Eating Guide and 60+ Recipes Inspired by Traditional Chinese Medicine to Calm the Mind and Achieve Optimal Health: http://bit.ly/summer-healthy-eating.

Healthy Eating: Autumn Healthy Eating Guide and 60+ Recipes Inspired by Traditional Chinese Medicine to Nourish the Skin and Achieve Optimal Health: http://bit.ly/autumn-healthy-eating.

Healthy Eating: Winter Healthy Eating Guide and 60+ Recipes Inspired by Traditional Chinese Medicine to Warm Up the Body, Nourish Your Skin, and Achieve Optimal Health: http://bit.ly/winter-healthy-eating.

To help you get a best deal to learn healthy eating in all four seasons, I've bundled these four books into one set at a discounted price. Make sure you grab this book instead of purchasing four books individually: http://bit.ly/seasonal-healthy-eating

In addition, as you have discovered in the recipe section, from time to time I have incorporated herbs as one of the key ingredients into different dishes. Chinese herbs are an important part of Traditional Chinese Medicine and, if used properly, can have very effective healing benefits.

If you are interested in knowing more about Chinese herbal therapy, you could check out my other book that gives you an introductory understanding of Chinese herbs and 10 herbs you could get started with: http://bit.ly/chinese-herbs.

As I told you at the introduction, I am constantly learning and updating my knowledge about TCM and Food Therapy. If you would like to get a free updated version of this book plus my personal insights, experiments, and learnings on the same topic along the way as well as a list of other bonuses, don't forget to subscribe to my mailing list: http://bit.ly/signup-for-bonuses.

I look forward to having you in the journey to explore the wonders of TCM and Food Therapy together with you.

Last but not least, if you like this book, I'd greatly appreciate it if you could leave me a review (http://bit.ly/food-as-medicine-review) at Amazon to help others discover the book, so that other people can benefit from the content as well.

To your ultimate health and beauty,

Tracy

Appendix A: Foods of Five Energies

(You can have a print-ready Word document of this appendix here: bit.ly/food-as-medicine-appendixes.*)*

Cold	Cool	Neutral	Warm	Hot
Sugarcane, chrysanthemum flower, bitter melon, lotus root, water chestnut, kudzu root, watermelon, banana, mulberry, kelp, lettuce, watercress, orange peel, octopus, crab, sprout, honeysuckle	Millet, wheat, Chinese barley, eggplant, cucumber, winter melon, cauliflower, broccoli, celery, mustard green, napa cabbage, spinach, lily bulb, pea, mung bean, pear, papaya, tea leaf, tofu, mushroom, needle mushroom	Brown rice, taro, sweet potato, potato, cabbage, carrot, red bean, peanut, kidney bean, pistachio, soy milk, grape, black sesame seed, black fungus, black rice, black bean	Chive, cilantro, onion, mint, lichi, peach, cherry, chestnut, pumpkin, sticky rice, red date, walnut, lobster, fish, lamb, chicken, coffee, alcohol, cigarette, hawthorn berry	Chili pepper, ginger, black pepper

Appendix B: Foods of Five Flavors

(You can have a print-ready Word document of this appendix here: bit.ly/food-as-medicine-appendixes.*)*

Sour	Sweet	Bitter	Pungent	Salty
Lemon, lime, tomato, pineapple, green apple, strawberry, orange, grapefruit, hawthorn berry, plum, mango, vinegar, grape	Papaya, pear, apple, honey, red date, mushroom, taros, sweet potato, potato, pumpkin, brown rice, wheat, black bean, red bean, soy bean, cherry, lotus seed, grape, corn, sugarcane, peanut, chestnut, beet	Bitter melon, tea leaf, coffee, lettuce, arugula, broccoli rabe, mustard green, turmeric	Garlic, ginger, chili pepper, onion, scallion, radish, horse-radish, Brussels sprout, curry	Seaweed, kelp, pork, crab, shrimp, Himalayan salt, miso paste

Appendix C: Foods of Five Colors

(You can have a print-ready Word document of this appendix here: bit.ly/food-as-medicine-appendixes.*)*

Red	White	Yellow	Green	Black
Red radish, red bell pepper, apple, cherry, watermelon, red chili pepper, red date, pomegranate, tomato, red bean, goji berry, cauliflower, strawberry, persimmon, pork, beef, lamb	Chinese yam, lily bulb, lotus root, lotus seed, Chinese barley, white radish, potato, tofu, white bean, white fungus, button mushroom, pear, water chestnut, taro, onion, garlic, egg, goat cheese, milk, white radish, white sesame seed, lichi, fish, chicken, almond, winter melon, whitebait, sticky rice, peanut	Ginseng, brown rice, quinoa, millet, sweet potato, pineapple, mango, pumpkin, papaya, lemon, chestnut, ginger root, turmeric, curry, buckwheat, teff, amaranth, walnut, chick pea, oat, chrysanthemum, orange, banana, corn, needle mushroom, bamboo shoot, grapefruit, soy bean, tangerine, egg yolk, carrot	Collard greens, broccoli, lettuce, mustard green, broccoli rabe, arugula, baby spinach, spinach, cabbage, sprout, green bell pepper, lime, kale, celery, asparagus, cucumber, green tea, mocha, scallion, cilantro, parsley, basil, thyme, rosemary, green pea, chive, avocado, kiwi fruit, Brussel sprout, bitter melon, water spinach, watercress	Black rice, black sesame seed, black fungus, black bean, seaweed, kelp, algae, blackberry, mulberry, eggplant, mushroom, dark purple grape, purple cabbage

151

Appendix D: Foods of Four Movements

(You can have a print-ready Word document of this appendix here: bit.ly/food-as-medicine-appendixes.*)*

Upwards	Outwards	Downwards	Inwards
Usually applying to foods with hot or warm energies, and foods with sweet or pungent flavors (see "Appendix A: Foods of Five Energies" and "Appendix B: Foods of Five Flavors" for reference). Examples: ginger, scallions, chili peppers, garlic, and horse-radishes		Usually applying to foods with cold or cool energies, and foods with bitter, sour, or salty flavors (see "Appendix A: Foods of Five Energies" and "Appendix B: Foods of Five Flavors" for reference). Examples: bitter melons, plums, and honeysuckle flowers	

Appendix E: Foods with Different Organic and Common Actions

(You can have a print-ready Word document of this appendix here: bit.ly/food-as-medicine-appendixes.*)*

Food	Good for What Organ(s)?	Common Actions
Chinese yam	Spleen, stomach, kidneys	Improving digestion, losing weight, lowering down blood lipid levels and blood sugar levels
Lotus seed	Spleen, kidneys, heart	Calming the mind, relieving insomnia and palpitation, treating diarrhea
Mustard greens	Lungs, stomach, kidneys	Reducing phlegm, relieving coughing, improving appetite, improving digestion, relieving constipation
Sesame seeds	Stomach, liver, kidneys	Promoting red blood cell growth, relieving dizziness, nourishing hair, lowering down blood sugar levels, nourishing the skin, slowing down aging process
Bitter melon	Heart, liver, spleen, lungs	Clearing summer heat, improving vision, lowering down blood sugar levels, healing acne breakouts, fighting fatigue, calming the mind, relieving thirst, losing weight, detoxifying the body
Cherry	Spleen, stomach, liver	Promoting red blood cell production, preventing anemia, improving immunity, improving brain functions, nourishing the skin, potentially helping remove wrinkles
Mung bean	Live, kidneys	Fighting bacteria, preventing bacteria growth, lowering down blood lipid levels, preventing cancer, healing acne breakouts, brightening up the skin, improving appetite, preventing and treating heat stroke in summer, detoxifying the body
Kelp	Liver, kidneys	Helping fight radiation, lowering down blood pressure, improving immunity, lowering down blood sugar levels, relieving swelling, preventing heart problems, nourishing hair and skin, losing weight, lowering down aging process, preventing cancer, relieving constipation
Taro	Stomach, kidneys, spleen	Improving appetite, bringing down inflammation, improving qi and energy flow inside the body, improving immunity, relieving constipation
Kudzu root	Lungs, stomach, spleen	Relieving thirst, detoxifying the body, relieving diarrhea

153

Food	Good for What Organ(s)?	Common Actions
Ginger	Heart, lungs, stomach, spleen	Relieving coughing, dealing with nausea, relieving bloating and constipation,
Goji berry	Liver, kidneys	Improving vision, slowing down aging process, fighting fatigue, preventing cancer,
Chestnut	Spleen, stomach, kidneys	Preventing heart problems, slowing down aging process, preventing and lowering down blood sugar levels, preventing osteoporosis
Watermelon	Heart, lungs, bladders, stomach, spleen, liver	Clearing summer heat, improving urinary flow, relieving thirst, calming the mind, nourishing and brightening up the skin, hydrating the body, nourishing hair
Mushroom	Liver, stomach	Improving immunity, preventing cancer, lowering down blood sugar and blood lipid levels, improving digestion, relieving constipation
Chinese barley	Spleen, lungs, kidneys	Brightening up the skin, healing acne breakouts, improving urinary flow, improving blood and energy flow inside the body, reducing swelling
Lotus root	Heart, kidneys, stomach, spleen, lungs	Calming the mind, slowing down aging process, improving digestion, relieving diarrhea, relieving constipation, enriching and producing blood, reducing bruises
Celery	Stomach, lungs, liver	Lowering down blood pressure, detoxifying the body, preventing cancer, relieving hangover, improving digestion, reducing swelling, improving urinary flow, brightening up the skin, calming the mind, relieving insomnia
Longan berry	Heart, spleen, stomach	Relieving palpitation and insomnia, nourishing the skin, slowing down aging process, enriching and nourishing blood
Red date	Spleen, stomach	Nourishing the skin, enriching and producing blood, slowing down aging process, brightening up the skin, fighting fatigue

Appendix F: Foods for Nine Body Types

(You can have a print-ready Word document of this appendix here: bit.ly/food-as-medicine-appendixes.)

Body Type	Symptoms	Recommended Foods
Yin deficiency	It is likely that you have dry skin, warm hands and feet, a red face, dry eyes, and dry stool. You easily get thirsty.	Black bean, black sesame, lily bulb, tofu, soy milk, pork, white fungus, black fungus, squid, sesame oil, tomato, grape, orange, tangerine, water chestnut, banana, apple, mulberry, sugarcane, clam, persimmon, duck's egg, duck *Moderate the intake of lamb, shrimp, chive, red chili pepper, scallion, and ginger.*
Yang deficiency	You tend to have cold hands and feet.	More sweet foods (e.g. brown rice, sweet potato, and potato) and pungent foods (e.g. garlic, ginger, and scallion) that give the body warm energies. Beside, also consider shrimp, walnut, and royal jelly. You can refer to "Food of Fiver Flavors" and "Food of Fiver Energies" for more options.
Qi deficiency	You constantly feel weak and tired and easily get sick.	Brown rice, millet, soy bean, white bean, snow pea, broad bean, potato, Chinese yam, sweet potato, mushroom, carrot, goose, lotus seed, chestnut, shrimp, eel, ginseng *Moderate the intake of buckwheat, grapefruit, raw white radish, orange, and water spinach.*
Qi depression	You easily get dark eye circles, and easily get bruises even you are only mildly hurt.	Oatmeal, cilantro, white radish, scallion, rose tea, garlic, onion, bitter melon, kelp, seaweed, algae, carrot, orange, tangerine, hawthorn berry *Meanwhile, make sure you get enough sleep and physical activities; and participate in group activities and stay connected.*
Blood stasis	You have acne-prone skin and may have bad breaths from time to time.	Seaweed, hawthorn berry, black bean, soy bean, mushroom, eggplant, mango, papaya, seaweed, kelp, algae, white radish, carrot, orange, tangerine, grapefruit, peach, plum, vinegar, rose pedal, green tea, mocha, brown sugar, wine *Moderate the intake of oily foods especially those with saturated fat from animals.*

Body Type	Symptoms	Recommended Foods
Dampness heat	You often feel depressed and suffer from insomnia.	Bitter melon, mung bean, mustard green, winter melon, cucumber, water spinach, watercress, watermelon, millet, Chinese barley, kudzu root, lotus seed, red bean, napa cabbage, celery, cabbage, purple cabbage, lotus root *Moderate the intake of walnut, lamb, goose, eel, cilantro, chili pepper, alcoholic beverage, oily and fried foods, foods prepared by hotpot, and barbecued foods.*
Phlegm dampness	You might be overweight and feel heavy in four limbs.	Winter melon, Chinese barley, seaweed, radish, scallion, garlic, kelp, seaweed, algae, olive, bamboo shoot, white radish, orange, horseradish, Chinese yam *Moderate the intake of red date, plum, persimmon, and sweet, oily, and sticky foods in general.*
Special diathesis	You easily get allergy and are sensitive to environmental changes.	A plant-based diet is recommended *Make sure you cut down the intake of alcoholic beverages, pungent foods, beef, goose, eggplant, chili pepper, coffee, strong tea, and seafood like shrimp, fish, and crab.*
Gentleness	You have a healthy and balanced body.	It is recommended you continue to have a well-balanced plant-based diet.

Appendix G: Food with Different Alkalinity and Acidity

(Italicized items are NOT recommended)

(You can have a print-ready Word document of this appendix here: bit.ly/food-as-medicine-appendixes.*)*

Most Alkaline	Moderately Alkaline	Mildly Alkaline	least Alkaline
Baking soda, sea salt, mineral water, umeboshi plum, pumpkin seed, *hydrogenated oil,* lentil, sweet potato, miso, onion, seaweed, sea vegetable, lime, nectarine, persimmon, raspberry, watermelon, tangerine, pineapple	Spices (e.g. cinnamon), valerian, soy sauce, molasses, cashew, chestnut, pepper, kohlrabi, parsnip, taro, garlic, asparagus, kale, parsley, endive, arugula, mustard green, ginger root, broccoli, grapefruit, citrus, olive, longanberry, mango, honeydew, cantaloupe	Most herbs (e.g. bergamot, chrysanthemum, lemongrass, echinacea, ephedra, and fevefew), green tea, mocha, rice syrup, apple cider vinegar, sake, quail egg, primrose oil, sesame seed, cod liver oil, almond, sprout, potato, bell pepper, mushroom, fungi, cauliflower, cabbage, ginseng, eggplant, pumpkin, collard greens, avocado, apple, pear, cherry, blackberry, peach, papaya	White willow bark, slippery elm, *sulfite,* ginger tea, umeboshi vinegar, algae, blue-green sea vegetables, human breast milk, oat, quinoa, wild rice, japonica rice, avocado oil, most seeds, coconut oil, olive/macadamia oil, linseed oil, flex oil, Brussel sprout, beet, chive, cilantro, celery, scallion, okra, cucumber, turnip greens, squash, lettuce, jicama, orange, apricot, banana, blueberry, pineapple, raisin, grape

least Acidic	mildly Acidic	Moderately Acidic	Most Acidic
Curry, *MSG*, *kona coffee*, honey, maple syrup, rice vinegar, cream, butter, yogurt, goat/sheep cheese, chicken egg, gelatin, organs, venison, fish, wild duck, triticale, millet, kasha, amaranth, brown rice, pumpkin seed oil, grape seed oil, sunflower oil, pine nut, canola oil, spinach, fava bean, kidney bean, black-eye pea, string bean, zucchini, chutney, coconut, pickled fruit, dry fruit, fig, persimmon juice, date	Vanilla, stevia, benzoate, alcohol, black tea, balsamic vinegar, cow milk, aged cheese, soy cheese, coat milk, lamb, shell fish, goose, turkey, buckwheat, wheat, teff, kamut, white rice, almond oil, sesame oil, safflower oil, tapioca, tofu, pinto bean, white bean, red bean, mung bean, chard, plum, prune, tomato	Nutmeg, *aspartame*, *coffee*, *saccharin*, *psychotropics*, milk protein, soy milk, pork, veal, mussel, squid, chicken, corn, rye, oat bran, pistachio seed, chestnut oil, *lard*, pecan, palm kernel oil, green pea, peanut, snow pea, legumes, carrot, chick pea, cranberry, pomegranate	Pudding, jam, jelly, *table salt*, beer, yeast, sugar, cocoa, white vinegar, *antibiotics*, processed cheese, ice cream, beef, lobster, barley, *processed flour*, *cottonseed oil*, hazelnut, walnut, Brazil nut, *fried food*, soybean, carob

158

Made in the USA
Lexington, KY
05 December 2016